The Beginner's Guide to the Eight Extraordinary Vessels

of related interest

Acupuncture for Surviving Adversity
Acts of Self-Preservation
Yvonne R. Farrell
ISBN 978 1 78775 384 6
eISBN 978 1 78775 385 3

Treating Emotional Trauma with Chinese Medicine
Integrated Diagnostic and Treatment Strategies
CT Holman, M.S., L.Ac.
ISBN 978 1 84819 318 5
eISBN 978 0 85701 271 5

Psycho-Emotional Pain and the Eight Extraordinary Vessels
Yvonne R. Farrell
ISBN 978 1 84819 292 8
eISBN 978 0 85701 239 5

Eight Extraordinary Channels – Qi Jing Ba Mai
A Handbook for Clinical Practice and Nei Dan Inner Meditation
Dr David Twicken DOM, LAc
ISBN 978 1 84819 148 8
eISBN 978 0 85701 137 4

The Beginner's Guide to the Eight Extraordinary Vessels

Mikschal (Dolma) Johanison, D.Ac., L.Ac.

Contributing Editor: Devon Gray, L.Ac., MAOM, Dipl.OM

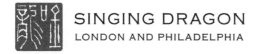
SINGING DRAGON
LONDON AND PHILADELPHIA

First published in Great Britain in 2022 by Singing Dragon,
an imprint of Jessica Kingsley Publishers
An Hachette Company

1

Copyright © Mikschal (Dolma) Johanison 2022

The right of Mikschal (Dolma) Johanison to be identified as the Author of the Work has been asserted by her in accordance with the Copyright, Designs and Patents Act 1988.

Front cover image source: Shutterstock®.

The information contained in this book is not intended to replace the services of trained medical professionals or to be a substitute for medical advice. The complementary therapy described in this book may not be suitable for everyone to follow. You are advised to consult a doctor before embarking on any complementary therapy programme and on any matters relating to your health, and in particular on any matters that may require diagnosis or medical attention.

A CIP catalogue record for this title is available from the British Library and the Library of Congress

ISBN 978 1 78775 831 5
eISBN 978 1 78775 832 2

Printed and bound by CPI Group (UK) Ltd, Croydon, CR0 4YY

Jessica Kingsley Publishers
Carmelite House
50 Victoria Embankment
London EC4Y 0DZ

www.singingdragon.com

In pursuit of my own personal excellence

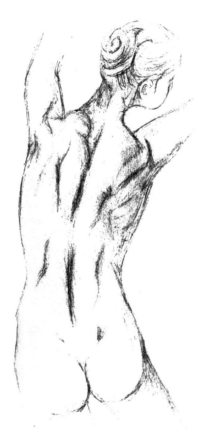

Drawing by Erin Stevenson

Contents

Acknowledgments

This book has been made possible with the help of many hands:

Erin Stevenson

Lil Kilgallen

Chris Tarbox

Janene Borandi

Nicole Asbahr

Thank you, ladies, for your contributions to this body of work.

Preface

This book intends to offer a different perspective on the eight extraordinary vessels. It is important to bear in mind that the theory of the eight extraordinary vessels has been adopted by practitioners over time and across the miles with varying opinions on how best to approach the employment and application of that theory. However, one thing that remains true is the value of the eight extraordinary vessels in the healing process. This book is designed for the novice regarding the application of the extraordinary vessels and offers a safe and basic approach.

The motivation for this manuscript is based on the works of Li Shi Zhen as translated by Miki Shima and Chuck Chase (Chase and Shima, 2010), the hands-on experience of Kiiko Matsumoto as witnessed in workshop format, and more than eleven years of clinical experience of using eight extraordinary treatments in everyday treatment planning.

CHAPTER 1

PRELIMINARIES

Healing patients requires practitioners to be competent and skillful at their trade. Part of being competent is embodying the history of theory and how theory becomes practice. Acupuncture history and culture is vast and dates back thousands of years. In fact, no one knows with certainty exactly when it began. Without honoring the history, competency becomes weak in the practitioner. It is the wisdom of past masters of the trade that has allowed modern-day practitioners to carry on the traditions of Eastern medicine. Who we are as healers is a reflection of the embodiment of acupuncture history, our own personal journey, and the interconnectedness we cherish with our healer ancestry.

The history is vast and has been in existence for thousands of years. In terms of dating the development of holistic medicine practices, the start date remains unknown, but many scholars suggest 2nd century CE, or perhaps even earlier. In the unfolding of the eight extraordinary vessel theory, the most recognized source is Li Shi Zhen, who, in the 16th century, made a thorough exposition of the eight extraordinary vessels and the herbal remedies that complement the effects of acupuncture. His understanding of the eight extraordinary pulses is unparalleled. In the 8th century, prior to the works of Li, a king and physician named Trisong Detsen greatly influenced holistic medicine. He taught about the deep energetic pathways of the point systems and how they are aligned with the "winds and channels" within the body. Further, he taught herbal remedies and moxibustion as the primary source of medicine. Trisong Detsen gathered practitioners from India, Tibet, Nepal, China, and the Turkic regions of Central Asia, who were all practicing medicine according to their cultures and lineage teachings. He encouraged the physicians to share ideas about the channels and points, winds, elements, and chakras within the body, and, further, to discuss practices and pathology. The meeting marked the beginning of integrative medicine and initiated a collective approach to medical practices with a holistic understanding.

The energetic channels comprise the oldest medical system in existence, which has been preserved and transmitted through turbulent global dynamics and across borders, cultures, and generations. Although the progression of Western medical technology has saved many lives, the best approach to medicine is informed by the successes of both the East and the West.

The Tibetan Medical System, one of the oldest medical systems in existence, dates to a time before the discovery of written language. Still preserved to this day are beautiful medical paintings that were created for Tibetan medical students to understand how diseases and health live in the body, including causes and conditions, consequences, and cures. The ancestors of this ancient medical system discovered points, channels, and elements that make up both human and animal bodies. This system offered herbal remedies and acupuncture, although needles were not used at that time; rather, the acupuncture points were palpated. Additionally, the Tibetan Medical System relied on bleeding, cupping, and moxibustion as cures for disease. The Chinese are also rightly given credit for these same practices still in existence today.

Miles apart, the Tibetans and Chinese were separately and simultaneously developing a medical system, discovering the energetic point system and deep pathways in the body. They were learning how pathology resides within these deep pathways and how that leads to disease. These scholars realized the healthier the channels, the healthier the human. It was during these early centuries that practitioners made the connection between the wellness of the channels and elements and a person's spiritual advancement; that is, the more physically balanced we are, the clearer the path to spiritual attainment. While many seek acupuncture for physical reasons, others seek it for its ability to broaden perspective and deepen spiritual connection.

In the 16th century, Li Shi Zhen, both a masterful physician and a prolific writer, completed several books; the most widely known is the *Compendium of Materia Medica*. His work regarding the eight extraordinary vessels came later, and in 2010 a translation was published by Charles Chase and Miki Shima, both licensed acupuncturists for many years and masters in their own right. Li first wrote about the eight extraordinary vessels through the lens of herbal medicine, and he blended treatment strategies by using both herbs and acupuncture in treating his patients. The translation of his work includes many of these treatment strategies.

Li was a physician, writer, spiritual advisor, and teacher. One of his main methods in relating his work was through direct transmission to other physicians (acupuncturists and herbal medicine practitioners). He kept volumes of medical journals regarding his work and discoveries, which became more controversial as his work evolved to connect physical, emotional, and spiritual health as interactive components of the human experience. In an increasingly temperamental political climate, the circumstances of Li's death became suspicious as many speculated that he was assassinated while walking home alone by two colleagues in an effort to cease the proliferation of his work.

The exact dates of the discovery and earliest uses of the eight extraordinary vessels remains contested. The vessel system was depicted in 8th-century paintings and there are teachings within Buddhist philosophy suggesting knowledge of the energetic meridian system of sentient beings dating before the common era. The consensus among most modern practitioners suggests that prior to the 11th century the extraordinary vessels were viewed as deep meridians not to be touched since they hold the sacred blueprints of a person's destiny.

Early practitioners and philosophers were not afraid to use these vessels. Li encouraged all of his students as herbalists and acupuncturists to honor and practice the highest level of medicine by incorporating these vessels into their treatments. In this way, he believed practitioners could serve the highest purpose.

The eight extraordinary vessels are viewed separately from the twelve primary channels, although the two meridian systems connect. Each extraordinary vessel consists of master and couple points, with many points on their respective trajectories located on the primary meridians. For example, the Yang Qiao Mai master point is Bladder 62 and its couple point Small Intestine 3. The names of the eight vessels changed over time, but since Li Shi Zhen's work, they are referred to as Chong Mai, Du Mai, Ren Mai, Dai Mai, Yin Wei Mai, Yang Wei Mai, Yin Qiao Mai, and Yang Qiao Mai.

Generally speaking, the eight extraordinary vessels hold the blueprint and consciousness of our lives. They record and store our memories from previous lives as well as events and experiences of this life. They have the capacity to unleash our potential, and to propel us to a higher state of being. Pathology can be stored in the extraordinary vessels, either from a previous life or current life, or from chronic patterns of disharmony within the twelve primary channels.

In modern scientific terms, we could relate the eight extraordinary vessels to the dynamic of nature versus nurture. They are the vault of possibilities and consequences alike. As practitioners, we understand that lifestyle choices accumulate day by day and these can be to the benefit or detriment of the existing genetic canvas.

Some practitioners have reported reluctance to treat patients on the extraordinary meridians. It is believed that accessing them is essentially accessing a patient's DNA and offers the prospect of going beyond superficial phenomena and symptoms. Thus, treating a patient on the deeper vessels can make a practitioner nervous; however, there is no need to be apprehensive when properly informed and trained. On the contrary, treating the extraordinary vessels can be a wonderfully affirming learning experience. The process should, however, be approached with reverence and great care.

The fear harbored by some practitioners regarding treatment of the eight extraordinary vessels has left many patients under-treated. It is a disservice to patients for budding practitioners to avoid using these vessels. Failing to harmonize the eight extraordinary vessels is like having gold stashed away and reaching the end of life without transforming those resources into a lasting legacy. As practitioners, we can guide others in dusting off their treasure maps and evolving toward the clearest expression of their gifts. The key is to develop confidence in treating these vessels. All patients at some point in their treatment plan develop the potential to be a candidate for treatment on the eight extraordinary vessels.

Because these vessels travel with the consciousness, going from lifetime to lifetime, a person cannot achieve their potential unless these vessels are open, functioning, and healthy. If there is pathology within the extraordinary vessels, a person cannot have full health. While a person may appear healthy in general and report a level of contentment with their life, ultimately they are not achieving their highest potential in health within the mind–body perspective.

Pathology can come from lifestyle (e.g., poor diet, lack of adequate exercise, negative habitual behaviors), genetics, traumatic experiences, emotional disturbances, or external pathogens such as cold and flu. Practitioners deal with these sorts of conditions every day in treating patients. This heavily populated world is full of viruses, diseases, genetically modified foods, and toxic chemicals and wavelengths. Family history may include any number of chronic health issues. Personal hygiene, lifestyle, and how well we take care of ourselves and the environment in which we live also impact our wellbeing. There is a host of environmental causes that lead to pathology and disease, including anything from verbal abuse to a war veteran's traumatic experiences.

Stress and trauma are associated with pathology. Most people experience multiple traumas to varying degrees throughout the course of their life. These traumas cannot be compared or measured because perceptions differ across populations and even within the context of one person's life. What causes post-traumatic stress disorder (PTSD) in one person may not cause it in another, depending on how each person perceives the environmental conditions in relation to their internal resources and awareness. Perceptions of trauma take root in the eight extraordinary vessels.

It is possible to avoid specific pathologies. A person born into a family with a history of heart disease or diabetes, for example, can make life choices that alter the probability of pathology manifesting. They can make decisions for the body, mind, and spirit that mitigate a pervasive genetic medical condition.

Given that we are complex beings, and everything is connected, there is an emotional component involved in every physical ailment. Whether we are suffering from a sports injury, chronic disease, or acute virus, the emotional component can be the piece of the puzzle that creates the greatest disharmony. The wound may heal physically, but unless the emotional component is addressed, the healing is incomplete, and other symptoms may arise. This is where the extraordinary vessels can shine as an approach to treatment, unleashing that which holds people back from achieving their highest potential.

Acupuncture practitioners use a channel and point system to address physical, emotional, and spiritual symptoms. This medicine creates the possibility for revelations to naturally unfold for the patient. It creates ease in the body, encouraging smooth channels for energy, blood, and spirit to flow unencumbered by disease.

Treating on the eight extraordinary vessels will strengthen the entire system on a physical, emotional, mental, and spiritual level. Treatments impact all levels of the body, and engage with all the meridians, to include the twelve primary channels. It is best to treat the eight extraordinary vessels and twelve primaries in tandem, whether applying an eight principle or five element constitutional approach. The best strategy is to plan for both the short and long term, which can be accomplished by applying these theories in tandem.

The extraordinary vessels are often referred to as seas or oceans. This is because they have a broader span of influence in the body on all three levels of existence (mind–body–spirit). In general terms, the eight extraordinary vessels strengthen the entire system and the associations between all the channels in the body. These vessels, when healthy, bring harmony to various axes in the body and stabilize a person's mind. However, they are prone to accumulating and creating excess in the body on physical and emotional levels.

Based upon an individual's karmic consequences, various illnesses can be stored or stagnated in the eight extraordinary vessels. The hereditary conditions a person is born with can be lodged in muscles, tendons, cells, and tissues. Using the eight extraordinary vessels, practitioners can access primordial energy which can unlock karmic memory and the set of conditions holding the patient back from overall health and wellbeing.

The eight extraordinary vessels hold our consciousness, or what many early philosophers refer to as "mind stream." When a person dies, any unresolved karma remains in the mind stream, and is present in the rebirth; this is what is meant by "stagnating in the eight extraordinary vessels." The pathological karma continues in the mind stream of the individual until it is resolved, purified, extinguished, or exhausted. Individuals can have multiple pathologies within the extraordinary vessels on all three levels of existence. The pathology within the extraordinary vessels is interdependent with the twelve primary meridians, meaning the pathology itself is not separated in the body, but rather impacts the entire network—yin and yang alike. Ideally, the practitioner will work on the twelve primaries and resolve as much as possible before treating the eight extraordinary vessels.

The twelve primary meridians do not traverse multiple lifetimes; rather, they begin and end with each physical body. The eight extraordinary vessels, however, remain intact energetically despite physical death. They are the thread of continuity that navigates the bardo states to be reincarnated in the following life, in a new physical form. Because each person has free will, karma will reflect the sum of one's choices. At death, the extraordinary vessels collect the karma from the most recent life and, ideally, the consciousness exits via the crown chakra.

According to classical texts, the consciousness travels for about 49 days in the bardo state prior to reincarnating. At the moment the consciousness is ready to manifest in the physical again, there is an opportunity to exercise free will regarding how the next life will manifest. The more awareness and spiritual attainment an individual was able to cultivate in the previous life, the more prepared the soul is to choose an advantageous vortex through which to manifest from the bardo.

The eight extraordinary vessels are the container of consciousness, carrying our karma from lifetime to lifetime. This helps explain why these vessels are seen as reservoirs with overflow and excess. As we move through the continuum of existence, we both collect and pacify karma. These karmic consequences rest in the eight extraordinary vessels. They shape our existence from one life to the next. At the moment of conception, the material body takes form and the twelve primary meridians come into physical existence. This helps explain why practitioners can address most symptoms with the twelve primary meridians. All phenomena arise from the five elements. Hence, five element acupuncture is extremely beneficial in addressing concerns on body, mind, and spirit levels, as each point on the body resonates with each level of existence. Phenomena are not only physiologically present, but include emotional and spiritual components, meaning each physiological condition has an emotional component to its reality.

Not all symptoms originate from the present lifetime. Because we enter each life with the karmic consequences of previous lives, we may experience symptoms that result from actions in a previous life. As we grow and develop in the present life, karma ripens and can manifest physically, emotionally, or spiritually, or as a combination. For example, a person in a previous life was a gladiator; although he may not have wanted to cause harm, for his own survival he had to hurt others, possibly take the life of another. As he enters the next life, there remains karmic consequence of his non-virtuous activity, which resides in the eight extraordinary vessels. The karmic consequence might manifest in this life as an unexplained shoulder or back injury; MRI images may show nothing is wrong physiologically, yet the pain does not permanently dissipate. Working on the twelve primary meridians will certainly help this patient in terms of pain management, but it may not be a long-term solution, especially if the root of the issue rests in one of the eight extraordinary vessels. The practitioner would need to access the extraordinary vessel in order to rid the patient of the pain permanently.

Merely activating the vessel is not sufficient to eliminate the pathology. The patient will begin to heal in such a way that they will address the karmic result of the pathology's origin, quite possibly without knowing exactly what is happening. As the practitioner begins to work on the vessel, the patient will change. Their perceptions and way of living will change; no matter how subtle it may seem, there will be change. The patient will begin to observe themselves getting better. The practitioner will be satisfied that qi and blood moved; something happened, and healing has occurred. However, what is happening is karma is being reconciled and is in the process of being pacified or ripened through a holistic approach.

If a person shows no physical sign of excess (e.g., in body shape, pulse, or tongue), they will have excess in another form, such as emotional or psychological conditions. These types of excess patterns will manifest on a continuum—for example, from mild depression to extreme states of mental illness. Excess in one of the eight extraordinary vessels is not necessarily seen in the same way as one might think of in an eight principle pattern of excess. For example, a person who has excess in the Yang Qiao Mai will display symptoms of depression, restlessness, feelings of being overwhelmed, some variation of sleep issues, significant nervous tension, and "secrets in their closet." They will have the perception of having done something wrong or being plagued on a daily basis by haunting emotions. In this condition, the pulses may seem normal, but are more oblong in shape; the tongue will be longer than most, more pointed, and perhaps slightly redder if heat is also present. Additionally, the tongue is described as having a "mountain top." This means that from a profile view the tongue will protrude up in the back and have a sharp descent distally. The tongue and pulse picture will not appear as in a typical damp or phlegm or excess condition presentation. The excess in this patient is more mental and emotional, and less physical. However, they will experience physical symptoms, such as pain in either shoulder or hip girdles, and it will run down the side of the body. They will be susceptible to headaches or sinus issues, or possibly both. Often, they will report issues with their eyes, either in vision problems, floaters, or generalized eye pain. Lastly, these patients most likely experience arthritic conditions from mild to more severe.

These indicators alone do not automatically equate to excess in the eight extraordinary vessels. To distinguish between excess in the extraordinary vessels and disharmony on one or two officials in the body takes time and skill on behalf of the practitioner. For the novice, a way of knowing is to treat the twelve primary meridians several times and evaluate progress. If the patient reports mild to no recovery, the pathology could be in an extraordinary vessel.

Because the physical body is a whole body with each part connecting to many other parts, these vessels intersect with one another as well as the twelve primary meridians. It is possible in the course of treating one of the eight extraordinary vessels that the root origin will present in a different extraordinary vessel. This is more common than most practitioners might realize. In this case, ideally the practitioner would finish the extraordinary series (discussed in Chapter 4) and return to the twelve primary meridians for a few treatments before moving to the next extraordinary vessel.

Some patients will require treatment on two or perhaps three extraordinary vessels over the course of time. The best treatment strategy is to focus on a rhythm of treating the twelve primary and eight extraordinary vessels in tandem. Occasionally, a pattern of disharmony will arise (e.g., cold or acute pain), and an eight principles approach is appropriate and helpful to the patient. Once the issue is resolved, simply return to the other work. It is possible to treat multiple extraordinary vessels simultaneously, but only if the practitioner is well trained in the theory. The practitioner needs to have a good understanding of how these vessels work both independently and interdependently in each unique individual.

Each extraordinary vessel is unique and responsible for different tasks in the body. The Chong Mai, Ren Mai, and Du Mai work closely together and are interwoven, albeit following different trajectories inside the torso of the body. The Dai Mai is the only vessel to traverse the body horizontally, wrapping around the girdle of the body and connecting with the Chong Mai, Ren Mai, and Du Mai. Within eight extraordinary vessel theory, the Chong Mai, Ren Mai, Du Mai, and

Dai Mai are distinguished as the four primaries of the eight extraordinary vessels (pairing is discussed in Chapter 12). The Yin Wei Mai and Yang Wei Mai work closely together and are considered the autobiography of our lives; they record our experiences and influence our behavior based upon those experiences. They follow vertical trajectories in the body. The Yin Wei Mai is found inferiorly, and the Yang Wei Mai is found on the sides of the body and travels through the shoulders to the side of the head (pairing is discussed in Chapter 12). The Yin Qiao Mai and Yang Qiao Mai also work closely together and are focused on the present moment of our lives: how we dance with the journey from birth to death in this particular life.

The eight extraordinary vessels are the holders of our consciousness and are interconnected. As we enter the current life, the vessels are in place; while the Chong Mai is instrumental in birth and the first few hours of life, the Chong Mai, Ren Mai, Du Mai, and Dai Mai are most active in the early stages of development following conception. They hold the karmic consequences that give us our shape, eyes, hair, gender, and so on. These genetic traits are a result of karmic consequences. The Yin Wei Mai, Yang Wei Mai, Yin Qiao Mai, and Yang Qiao Mai begin to work as soon as the baby enters the world from the womb. They work together and interconnect with the Chong Mai, Ren Mai, Du Mai, and Dai Mai. This is a very natural and fluid process in the body.

All beings die with karmic consequences of a particular life, as well as karma from previous lives that was not addressed in the current life. This is an expression of cyclic existence. The virtuous deeds as well as the collection of negative actions committed in a given life will ripen in the next. Therefore, each life is an opportunity to bring as much benefit as possible, not only for oneself but for the sake of those we love and care about.

Ren Mai is an extraordinary vessel, not to be confused with the Conception Vessel (CV), just as Du Mai does not refer to the Governor Vessel (GV). Ren Mai and Du Mai are different vessels operating on a different network from the CV and GV meridians. It is helpful to use the proper language within the context of the theory. In eight extraordinary vessel theory, the Chong Mai is also known as the Central Channel in the body. All eight vessels operate in broader pathways than the twelve primaries in the body and cover more areas. For example, the Yang Qiao Mai travels along the side of the body, impacting the entire lateral aspect of the lower limbs, shoulders, neck, and head. The Chong Mai impacts the midline and covers approximately two cun from the midline in each direction, including the Kidney meridian. This is another reason why Chong Mai trajectory points are on the Kidney meridian. The Dai Mai impacts all eight extraordinary vessels and twelve primaries, which further demonstrates how broadly the extraordinary vessels affect the network. Essentially, treating the Dai Mai has an impact on the entire system in the body as it binds all the meridians. The practitioner will want to keep this in mind during treatment planning and strategies.

One of the more common questions is when to start working with these vessels in the course of treatment. As a general rule, treating the eight extraordinary vessels is beneficial when there are (1) problems on more than one of the twelve primary meridians, (2) complicated or chronic conditions, (3) neurological conditions, (4) significant mental and/or emotional afflictions, and (5) patients who are elite athletes or performing artists (e.g., dancers, musicians). Only two or more of these descriptors are needed to make the decision. However, everyone benefits from being treated on the eight extraordinary vessels because we all have both positive and negative karma which leads to various conditions that may not have a conventional medicine label.

Number 5 above refers to children or adults who are engaged in high-pressure athletics or performing arts, such as Olympic or aspiring Olympic athletes, or advanced dancers or musicians. It is important to note the patient's perspective regarding the level of stress or pressure in their athletic or performance pursuits. People who feel they are under pressure to perform suffer from high levels of performance anxiety, and this type of anxiety over time affects the Yin Wei Mai, Yang Wei Mai, Yin Qiao Mai, and Yang Qiao Mai. A practitioner can help these patients maintain the activity they love doing, without suffering the consequences of performance anxiety, by treating the eight extraordinary vessels.

In terms of karma, karmic conditions, and cyclic existence, one does not need to believe in these concepts in order to treat and/or benefit from an eight extraordinary vessel treatment. It is important to bear in mind the many benefits of using these vessels as part of the overall treatment strategy and not become overly focused on the historical significance or concepts that incorporate a different perspective of life after death.

CHAPTER 2

THEORETICAL CONSIDERATIONS

During the process of intense learning about the eight extraordinary vessels, ideally the practitioner receives treatment on these vessels. It is important for practitioners to cultivate their own internal alchemy. It is not in the spirit of the eight extraordinary "lineage" to treat these vessels on patients and the practitioner not partake of their benefit during the course of learning. The great masters of the past were willing to work on the ties that bind us to cyclic existence; therefore, in deciding to treat patients on these deep pathways, one must not activate for others what one is not willing to do for oneself. Eight extraordinary vessels theory is rooted in Daoist, Buddhist, and Shamanic practices. Although not everyone may subscribe to these specific belief systems, everyone can benefit from eight extraordinary treatments. The masters advised that in working with these vessels, the practitioner becomes assistant to the patient's journey of spiritual cultivation.

Internal alchemy is interwoven with the eight extraordinary vessels. The theory suggests that learning about these vessels helps a patient to fulfill their potential. Taking the time to understand what the eight extraordinary vessels offer can be beneficial for both patient and practitioner. Working with energetic channels and channel systems has been recorded for thousands of years through various means. In order to fully experience internal alchemy, one needs to cultivate an understanding of the energies within the framework of the body through the use of breathing techniques, yoga, and meditation. The great benefits of working with the extraordinary vessels include the expansion of the breath, increased energy within the body, enhancement of the chakra system, and increased longevity. The medicinal perspective is interwoven with the spiritual perspective.

Internal alchemy emerges differently for different people. It is a process based on the individual's ability to cultivate spiritual awareness. While there are varying forms, meditation is crucial to a person's achievement in reaching the highest potential possible. This is because it allows one to gain a sense of spaciousness and awareness of what is happening on the inside and outside of the body. What is happening inside the body is a result of what is happening in the mind—meaning we can create our own reality. Longevity is desirable as it allows ample time for a person to address personal karmic work before dying and moving to the next life. Whether practitioner or patient, in the process of spiritual alchemy, achieving stillness, quietude, and a sense of enlightenment is important. This in turn heals the body and allows for a better quality of life.

We are in a complete state of homeostasis when the eight extraordinary vessels are in balance and the mind is stable. The goal of the practitioner is to help the patient achieve a state of equanimity, which requires the practitioner to also have a willingness to work on internal alchemy.

All of the extraordinary vessels should be thought of as vast meridians in the body, like seas or oceans rather than narrow channels such as creeks and rivers. They reach areas in the body as thick bands, binding the body, mind, and spirit together to make a complete whole. It is advised to treat the twelve primary vessels first for several treatments unless there is an acute situation. However, it is generally thought of as safe to treat the extraordinary vessels early in treatment, most especially the Yin Qiao Mai, Yang Qiao Mai, Yin Wei Mai, and Yang Wei Mai. It is recommended to wait to treat the extraordinary primaries (Chong Mai, Ren Mai, Du Mai, and Dai Mai) until much later in the overall treatment strategy. This harmonic state of being and strength is accomplished by treating the twelve primaries and the Qiao Mai and Wei Mai before treatment of the primaries contained within the eight extraordinary vessels. Imagine the Qiao Mai and Wei Mai as the structure, and the Chong Mai, Ren Mai, Du Mai, and Dai Mai as the pieces inside the structure. The practitioner would want the structure to be solid and stable prior to working on the inside pieces in order to provide the necessary support while internal alchemy is taking place.

—— CHAPTER 3 ——

PROCEDURE

In order to fully activate an extraordinary vessel, both the master and couple point need to be used. Without needling both the master and couple points, the meridian is not fully activated in the tradition of the extraordinary vessel theory. Using only the master point is not sufficient to fully engage the meridian according to the classical texts.

For males, the master point (MP) is on the left and couple point (CP) is on the right. For females, the master MP is on the right and CP is on the left.

When using trajectory points, open the MP and respective CP, then needle trajectory points bilaterally, usually using the long tonification technique.

Pairing extraordinary vessels means to activate two separate vessels simultaneously. This is not something a new practitioner should attempt until they have acquired knowledge, clinical experience, and a detailed understanding of how each vessel functions independently from the other vessels. Li Shi Zhen discussed pairings in his exposition more as a reflection of his findings in clinical practice. His clinical work brought to light how the extraordinary vessels function in health and disease. His exposition outlines the functional relationship between the vessels independently as well as when paired (Li Shi Zhen, cited in Chase and Shima 2010). The dynamics of paired vessels are outlined with more detail in Chapter 12. In more general terms, vessel pairing can be of value concerning certain conditions and/or in unique cases. However, it is recommended that pairing not occur too soon in treatment and only when the practitioner has acquired adequate knowledge of the vessels. When deemed appropriate to pair vessels, needle the MP and CP of each vessel separately (e.g., when pairing the Chong Mai and Ren Mai, open the MP and CP of Chong Mai first, and then open the MP and CP of Ren Mai). Again, more detailed information about pairing is discussed in Chapter 12.

There are varying opinions regarding how long needles should remain inserted. As a general rule, 20–40 minutes is acceptable, with 30 minutes at minimum being optimal. Ideally, the patient will come for treatment once a week for three weeks without a break. This is optimal in order to fully activate the vessel. If the patient cannot come every week for three weeks, then they should be treated at least every two weeks until the sessions are completed. A standard course of treatment might develop like this:

> Patient visits a total of three times, with one week in between treatments. The practitioner has made the decision to activate the Yin Wei Mai based on the diagnostic protocol. During the first treatment of the series of three, the MP and CP are the only two points used. During the second treatment, the MP and CP are opened and two or three points on the trajectory are needled bilaterally. On the last treatment of the series of three, the practitioner uses the MP, CP, and two to four points bilaterally on the trajectory.

A series of three treatments with a natural progression of adding trajectory points is a safe and beneficial method for the novice to begin learning how best to treat the eight extraordinary vessels. Generally, the MP and CP are not combined with the use of moxa; however, trajectory points can be treated in combination with moxa should the practitioner deem it appropriate.

Although unusual, there can be cases in which points off the trajectory are used during the course of extraordinary vessel treatments. Off-trajectory points are mentioned in Chapter 5 when discussing the vessels and their respective trajectory points.

Regarding needle retention time, the 30-minute rule is optimal. Activating these vessels can require the patient to engage in deep emotional work, so sufficient time must be allotted for the process. The patient needs to have stability in between treatments, so it is important for practitioners to allow ample time for the patient to acclimate to the activation of these vessels. Evidence suggests that treating according to the classical theory will not put the patient at risk emotionally. The treatments are powerful, and the impact on each patient is different and unpredictable. Leaving the needles in for 30 minutes yields a gentler and slower effect.

Time constraints of the past were not the same as time constraints of the present. A good rule of thumb is to have the patient retain the needles no less than 20 minutes and no more than an hour. If needles are not allowed to stay inserted for a full 30 minutes, the 20-minute rule will work, but the vessel may need to be activated more than allowed by the three-week series method. The 20-minute rule may work best for some patients who need a slower pace for deeper work.

Please consider that the practitioner is manipulating a patient's constitutional platform (chakra system). As mentioned above, it is important to set the stage for the patient to experience stability in the face of potentially challenging emotional work. Therefore, there is no need to lift, thrust, or twist the needles when treating the eight extraordinary vessels. Needle technique needs to be gentle and without action for the MP and CP, allowing the wisdom of the body to make its best decision. Therefore, the MP and CP should simply be needled with an "even technique" (i.e., no needle action). These vessels are dynamic enough on their own with a simple insertion of the needle to fen depth. Hence, the adage "less is more."

TRAJECTORY POINTS

The points we use to treat the extraordinary vessels are not part of the vessel itself; rather, they are merely the access points whereby practitioners gain entry to these vessels.

Points on the respective trajectories are needled bilaterally. It is acceptable and appropriate to perform a slight tonification or sedation needle technique on trajectory points in cases where the practitioner has deemed the patient deficient or in excess, respectively. Similarly, moxa can be applied to trajectory points only.

Trajectory points can be beneficial during the course of the extraordinary vessel treatments to treat specific conditions, whether physical, mental, or emotional. It is advised to add trajectory points gradually in order not to overwhelm the patient's energetic body.

Practitioners may approach the selection of trajectory points in the same manner as they would when employing a theory outside of the eight extraordinary model. However, within the context of the extraordinary treatments, the trajectory points do have an added meaning.

The intention with trajectory points is to enhance the energetic system beyond the master and couple points of the extraordinary vessel, regardless of which vessel is being treated. Trajectory points on the extraordinary vessel maintain their integrity and function according to any theory employed by the practitioner; however, when used in the context of one of the extraordinaries, they are magnified and take on a more spiritual role, depending upon which meridian and point is selected. For example, Kidney 9 is a wonderful point for building, nourishing, and supporting the Kidney meridian in general. When used in the context of an eight extraordinary treatment, it takes on the role of deepening the intrinsic wisdom of the patient.

Please refer to the trajectory point indications listed for each of the corresponding extraordinary vessels for more in-depth information.

Off-trajectory points can be used in advanced eight extraordinary treatments. It is best to use trajectory points on the targeted extraordinary vessel for at least the first three treatments. Once this has been completed, the practitioner may deem it beneficial to treat the vessel again, at which point it is generally safe to add points that are not on one of the eight extraordinary vessels, or a trajectory point from one of the other seven extraordinary vessels, but not the one being opened. A skilled practitioner with experience using these vessels will begin to understand how to discern between the points over time.

As mentioned previously, off-trajectory points can be used in rare cases, and some possibilities are offered in this book in the trajectory points indications sections. For those new to the theory, it is not advised to use off-trajectory points. It is more beneficial to the patient for the practitioner to become well versed in the theory before using them.

IN SUMMARY

First treatment: MP, CP only

Second treatment: MP + CP + 2–3 trajectory points

Third treatment: MP + CP + 2–4 trajectory points

In advanced treatments, Triple Burner points can be added to assist in energetic communication throughout the body (this is discussed more thoroughly in Chapter 7).

The eight extraordinary vessels are represented as overarching regulators of yin and yang and, by extension, the modulators of the rest of the channel system. Despite their close associations with the rest of the channels, the eight extraordinary vessels maintain a degree of autonomy. However, each extraordinary vessel exerts its own influence on every channel to some extent, and no single extraordinary vessel may be conceptualized in relation to any one primary channel. Chronic diseases ultimately afflict the extraordinary vessels, and over time excess conditions can accumulate within the system of the eight extraordinary vessels. There can be a mix of excess and deficiency conditions within these vessels in an individual. Even relatively minor deficiencies of the extraordinary vessels tend to reflect significant compromise in health.

Li Shi Zhen indicates in his work on the extraordinary vessels that the more profound and important role of the vessels is in relation to spiritual cultivation. In terms of internal alchemy, essence qi also refers to the "primordial qi of the cosmos." Essence qi originates from the Kidneys, and essence qi is necessary in order to undertake spiritual cultivation. When a person is "burning the candle at both ends," they are depriving themselves of the highest potential of spiritual cultivation because of the draining of essence qi. In order to achieve our highest spiritual potential, it is imperative that essence qi is not compromised.

It is important to remember physical conditions are not separate from spiritual deficiency. Spiritual deficiencies will manifest in the body physically at some point in a person's growth cycle. Internal cultivation cannot take place in a vacuum. The idea of running away and hiding in a cave can sound appealing to some; however, it is only through direct experience that we can ultimately grow internally and fulfill our lives' work in the present life. Otherwise, we are simply hiding out.

CHAPTER 4

DIAGNOSTIC PROTOCOLS

The procedure for diagnosis is generally determined by tongue, pulses, behavior, lifestyle, constitutional nature, signs, and symptoms.

Contained within the vessel description as outlined in this book, there are general ways of approaching the overall treatment strategy using the eight extraordinary vessels. Ideally, as a beginner a simple protocol would be used until the practitioner becomes more comfortable with the theory and develops a deeper understanding of the vessels.

A simple protocol begins with the Yin Qiao Mai and Yang Qiao Mai, followed by the Yin Wei Mai and Yang Wei Mai.

Simple protocol for treating vessels one by one
Yin Qiao Mai x 3
Followed by
Yang Qiao Mai x 3
Followed by
Yin Wei Mai x 3
Followed by
Yang Wei Mai x 3

Yin Qiao Mai and Yang Qiao Mai vessels can be paired (see Chapter 12 for more information), and Yin Wei Mai and Yang Wei Mai vessels can be paired if the patient is emotionally stable and has a support structure in place (i.e. family, friends and contact with community that would recognize any need for intervention while the patient is in long-term treatment). Typically, the practitioner treats each vessel a total of three times before moving to the next vessel. Should the practitioner decide to pair either the Qiao Mai or Wei Mai vessels, each pairing would be done a total of three times before moving to the next vessel.

Protocol for treating paired vessels

Yin Qiao Mai and Yang Qiao Mai x3

Followed by

Yin Wei Mai and Yang Wei Mai x3

After the Qiao Mai and Wei Mai vessel have been treated successfully, the practitioner can begin to work on the four primaries of the eight extraordinary vessels (Ren Mai, Du Mai, Chong Mai, and Dai Mai).

The practitioner may need to break from the extraordinary vessel treatments or stop pairing the vessels if the patient is feeling overwhelmed or becomes emotionally unstable. If the patient becomes emotionally distraught and/or overwhelmed, continue treating the vessel but stop the pairing of both yin and yang, and treat each vessel independently: Yang Qiao Mai, Yin Qiao Mai, Yang Wei Mai, Yin Wei Mai, respectively. Should the practitioner feel at any point that the patient is emotionally unstable, the practitioner should stop the treatments and return to the twelve primaries to support the person. Kidney and Spleen points are always beneficial in returning the patient to stable ground, and if appropriate Heart and/or Pericardium points can be treated to stabilize shen. It would be beneficial if the practitioner and patient determine they can resume the extraordinary treatments within a two-week period. However, it is especially important to monitor the patient closely.

Time between treatments varies based on the individual patient. However, under ideal circumstances the patient would receive three treatments within three weeks. After a short break between vessels, the practitioner can start on the next set of extraordinary vessel treatments.

After treating the Qiao Mai and Wei Mai, the practitioner can begin treatment on one of the four primaries of the eight extraordinary vessels. The recommended sequence options are as follows:

- Chong Mai, Ren Mai, Du Mai, Dai Mai

- Ren Mai, Du Mai, Chong Mai, Dai Mai

- Du Mai, Ren Mai, Chong Mai, Dai Mai

As a rule, Ren Mai and Du Mai are always consecutive in treatment, and the Dai Mai is always treated last. Chapter 13 explains in more detail about the Ren Mai and Du Mai relationship and why they would not be separated during the course of treatment. They may be paired but generally are not; only treat one vessel at a time before starting the next. While the primaries *can* be paired, it is recommended that each primary vessel be treated independently of the others.

Latent conditions may manifest during the course of treatment on the extraordinary vessels. Conditions must be expressed as they clear from the body, mind, and spirit. In these cases, the practitioner should continue with the established course of treatment as per the protocol.

Starting with the Qiao Mai and systematically working through the vessels in a specific order is recommended but not necessary. Should circumstances or conditions require a different approach, it would be wise to consider the risks. The main reason for using the systematic approach of treating the Qiao Mai, Wei Mai, and primary vessels in sequential order as noted above is that it is a more conservative and gentle approach for the beginner. Treating the Qiao Mai and Wei Mai first is a method of treating the physical body (container) first, thereby ensuring that it is stable enough to withstand the clearing and healing of the primaries. To compare it to building a house, it is a way of ensuring that the foundations, walls, and roof are in good order before renovating the inside with new paint, floors, and furniture.

There are cases of treating the primaries first. This does not, however, indicate an absence of pathology in the Qiao Mai and Wei Mai, and in all likelihood the practitioner would have to treat these vessels at some point during the course of the treatment strategy in the long term.

Reasons to jump protocol and skip the Qiao Mai and Wei Mai include infertility, acute emotional or mental distress such as suicide attempts, or, the contrary, a person who is doing well and has healthy Qiao Mai and Wei Mai. To determine the health of the Qiao Mai and Wei Mai, consider a patient's self-esteem and ability to adapt to change in addition to physical symptoms.

With healthy Qiao Mai, the patient is pleased with who they are, and they feel free to be spontaneous, capable of dancing with life gracefully, and can take what comes their way, navigating emotions in a healthy manner. With healthy Wei Mai, the patient is able to live fully in the present moment, not focusing on the past or living in the future (obsessive about future decisions); rather, they are comfortable living in the present moment, seeing it as a precious time. Further, they are generally optimistic, and able to see the benefit or lessons in each moment, no matter the circumstance. The patient's musculoskeletal structure is in good health and condition. Should the patient have one physical structure concern, it is wise to start on the Qiao Mai, or if there is one internal issue such as fatty liver or digestive issues, it is wise to treat the Wei Mai first. Nutrition is essential to the healthy communication between the Qiao Mai and Wei Mai. Food cravings, sensitivities, and allergies provide information about the conditioning of these vessels.

If the patient meets the criteria set for healthy Qiao Mai and Wei Mai, treating the four primaries initially is generally not a problem. However, if there is pathology in the Qiao Mai and/or Wei Mai, the patient is better served by receiving treatment according to the established protocol.

In treating the eight extraordinary vessels, just as with eight principle or five element theories, it is crucial to keep the course of treatment patient-centered. In practice, this requires continuous observation and re-evaluation of the patient and the feedback they provide regarding their experience from one treatment to the next. Lastly, one way to think about the interdependence of the Qiao Mai and Wei Mai is seeing the Qiao Mai as the "structure" and the Wei Mai as the guts inside the structure—the mushy gushy.

CHAPTER 5

THE VESSELS

QIAO MAI AND WEI MAI

The Qiao Mai are related to the left and right sides of the body, whereas the Wei Mai are related to the interior and exterior of the body. Although the trajectories for both the Qiao Mai and Wei Mai are similar and often paired with one another, in the beginning of treatment planning it is best to pair the Qiao Mai (Yin and Yang) before starting the Wei Mai, which are also generally paired (Yin and Yang).

PLEASE NOTE

The Qiao Mai are generally the only vessels where moxa is acceptable on the master and couple points. Moxa can be used on the *trajectory* points of all eight extraordinary vessels; however, generally speaking, only the Qiao Mai master and couple points should be treated with moxa.

The Qiao Mai govern the present moment, whereas the Wei Mai govern the recordings of our lives, continually gathering data and creating our autobiographies. The Wei Mai can be visualized as pearls on a string, lifetime after lifetime—the broader picture of multiple lifetimes. Li Shi Zhen wrote in his notes that he often started with the Qiao Mai in the course of treatments in order to help the patient process current events in their life before moving forward with addressing past-life karmic consequences that were ripening in the patient's current life. His intention in treating this way afforded the patient a more gradual and holistic healing process.

While there is no real consensus on which vessel to start with in treating patients, most experienced eight extraordinary vessel practitioners would agree starting on either Qiao Mai or Wei Mai is most beneficial before starting with one of the four primaries (Chong Mai, Ren Mai, Du Mai, and Dai Mai). The Qiao Mai and Wei Mai work closely together; that which is happening in the patient's current life is a reflection of what has happened in previous lives. This life will have an impact on the next life and so on. The Qiao Mai and Wei Mai work in tandem to create continuity and track karmic ties over lifetimes of experience.

In terms of procedure there are a few acceptable options. Treatment begins with Yin Qiao Mai, and after the course of three consecutive treatments the practitioner moves to the Yang Qiao Mai for three consecutive treatments. The practitioner can start with the Yang and then move to the Yin if deemed more beneficial to the patient. Trajectory points can be used, starting with the first treatment. There is no need to wait to use trajectory points until the second treatment as is practiced with the four primaries. Additionally, there is no need to shift to the twelve primaries in between treating the Qiao Mai.

Treatment can also begin with pairing the Yin and Yang Qiao Mai. The practitioner would open the master point, then the couple point on the Yin Qiao Mai; they would then open the master point on the Yang Qiao Mai followed by its couple point. After each vessel has been activated, the practitioner chooses one or two trajectory points either on the Yin or the Yang Qiao Mai, or one of each. Pairing treatments are also done in three consecutive treatments at minimum.

After treating the Qiao Mai, whether one at a time or paired, the practitioner can move directly to the Wei Mai, and follow the same procedure as conducted with the Qiao Mai. After the Qiao Mai and Wei Mai have been treated, the practitioner would shift to the twelve primary vessels for approximately four to five treatments before moving on to an extraordinary primary vessel.

Some practitioners have had success pairing Yin Qiao Mai with Yin Wei Mai, and pairing Yang Qiao Mai with Yang Wei Mai, but one would not normally pair Yin Qiao Mai with Yang Wei Mai or Yin Wei Mai with Yang Qiao Mai. Ideally, the pairings would be one of the following:

- Yin Qiao Mai with Yang Qiao Mai

- Yin Wei Mai with Yang Wei Mai

- Yin Qiao Mai with Yin Wei Mai

- Yang Qiao Mai with Yang Wei Mai

The Qiao Mai and Wei Mai are consistently addressing the yin and yang energies. The vessels penetrate the brain physically and have significant impact spiritually. There is a deeper trajectory that wraps around the eye and connects to the Bladder meridian at acupuncture point Bladder 1. Note that this particular trajectory impacts the brain and head.

Li Shi Zhen noted the Qiao Mai are often treated specifically for their ability to direct patients toward spiritual development, addressing and working within the spiritual body. The day-to-day functions of the Qiao Mai are important on all levels, especially as they relate to the diurnal transmission and regulation of yin and yang, synthesizing protective qi and nutritive qi. Consider the theory in practical terms by reviewing the circadian rhythms: hormones, circulation, body temperature, bowel movements, eating, and so on. These natural day-to-day functions are primarily governed by the Qiao Mai.

> The Wei and Qiao Mai Vessels are best understood as two functional pairs, devoted to regulating the yin and yang in relatively superficial expression of qi, even as they are grounded in deeper reserves of vitality within the body. (Li Shi Zhen, cited in Chase and Shima, 2010, p.30)

The Yin Qiao Mai governs the primal qi in a person and has a strong connection and placement in the progression of internal alchemy. The Qiao Mai are paramount in the functioning of the eight extraordinary vessels as a system. The Qiao Mai hold importance not only in physiology but in one's ability to expand spiritually as well. If a person is spiritually deprived (often described as "lost"), the practitioner can address this deficiency through the Qiao Mai.

The Qiao Mai and Wei Mai travel from head to toe, and, as mentioned before, work closely together energetically. The relationship between the Yin Wei Mai and Yin Qiao Mai in the chest enables a person to recover from traumas of the heart and to speak from the heart. The Yin Qiao Mai facilitates this healing within the Yin Wei Mai.

The Yin Wei Mai relates to all the faculties of yin, from the inside out. Again, the Wei Mai energetically function from within to without, and the Qiao Mai, from side to side. In treating the Qiao Mai and Wei Mai, the practitioner covers the entire human body at all three levels of existence (physical, mental/emotional, and spiritual).

Li Shi Zhen suggests in his personal notes that the practitioner is not serving patients unless at some point in the overall treatment strategy the eight extraordinary vessels are recruited. He believed the Qiao Mai have more to do with cultivating internal alchemy, playing a critical role in the cultivation process in one lifetime. They are related to the way a person dances with life, navigating what is confronted in a single lifetime. A person's reactions to the unfolding of life, whether accepting or denying, embracing, or pushing away are largely governed by the health and vitality of the Qiao Mai.

YIN QIAO MAI

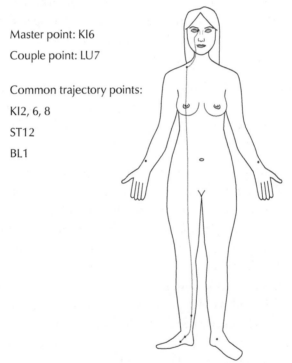

Master point: KI6

Couple point: LU7

Common trajectory points:

KI2, 6, 8

ST12

BL1

Figure 5.1 Yin Qiao Mai (Yin Heel Vessel)

Master Point: Kidney 6

Couple Point: Lung 7

The Yin Qiao Mai fosters destiny and allows for the cultivation of inner strength and faith, to be able to get through the hardest moments in one's current life. Because the Qiao Mai and Wei Mai function interdependently, the Yin Qiao Mai generates healing of disease or trauma that has affected the Yin Wei Mai. The root origin of pathology may lie in the Yin Qiao Mai and will impact the Yang Qiao Mai because they are interdependent. In the same way, healing in one vessel may spur healing in another. Think in terms of yin and yang when thinking of the Qiao Mai and Wei Mai. Together, they mobilize consciousness for the purpose of self-reflection and meditation, especially the Yin Qiao Mai. Additionally, it is this particular vessel that supports and sustains self-regard, allowing for an authentic life. The Qiao Mai and Wei Mai are nearly impossible to separate in terms of how they function in the body. However, there are a few characteristics quite specific to the Yin Qiao Mai.

The Yin Qiao Mai is about the physical holding of the body (e.g., holding muscles to tissue, holding the frame upright, holding organs in place). It is similar to the theory regarding the functions of the Spleen official in five element theory. Specifically, the Yin Qiao Mai is responsible for holding the muscles, tissues, and the skeletal system, keeping the eyes in the head, and for the integrity of the self in terms of walking one's path, which includes possessing a level of self-honesty and integrity in service of living authentically. When there is discomfort or pathology with the true self or one's integrity is not intact, one may experience a lack of interest in being in the world. When this happens, the person is no longer motivated and begins to give up on life.

The emotions most pronounced with Yin Qiao Mai pathology include issues of self-trust, abandonment, severe depression, low self-esteem, self-destructive behavior, and feelings of unworthiness. These emotions are measured against a continuum, meaning they can be very subtle to more extreme cases.

PLEASE NOTE ——————————————

There is a specific protocol used within the eight extraordinary vessel theory that addresses concerns of suicidal ideation. This is discussed in the section pertaining to pairing techniques.

Specific to Yin Qiao Mai disharmony, the patient experiences nightmares, insomnia, deep sadness, and depression, and is unable to enjoy life no matter what fortunate circumstances exist. There could be alcoholism currently or in the past, and anxiousness associated with a deep, deep fear. This vessel intersects with the Chong Mai. Therefore, it can be used to treat physical symptoms relating to low back pain, genital pain, and any disharmonies associated with the pelvic cavity. In fact, it would be more beneficial to treat the Yin Qiao Mai prior to treating the Chong Mai. Naturally, the Yin Qiao Mai also intersects with its sister, the Yang Qiao Mai.

The Yin Qiao Mai travels into the brain and is associated with energetic imbalances pertaining to left and right issues, one-sided pain and/or problems with gait, inversion of the foot, osteoporosis, pain in the eyes, tumors and cysts, hypothyroidism, and autoimmune disorders.

Yin Qiao Mai and the Yang Qiao Mai allow for a vital, powerful, and graceful dancing movement, engendering an elegant flow with the constantly changing energies and emotions in life. Harmony of the Qiao Mai vessels allows for the natural course of destiny with inner strength and faith in oneself. This harmony supports the transcendence of adversity into physical, emotional, and spiritual success.

Trajectory Points

Kidney 2, 8, 11–27

Stomach 1, 2, 3, 4, 9, and 12

Bladder 1

Gallbladder 20

KIDNEY 2

- Clears empty heat from Kidneys (night sweats, restless feet)

- Cools the blood

- Regulates kidneys (genital issues, kidney stones) and lower jiao (lower extremity pain)

- Moistens throat; clears painful obstruction in throat

- Invigorates Yin Qiao Mai

- Unfreezes ice and softens water; makes channel more fluid and vibrant

- Allows for self-expression—Yin Qiao Mai specifically

- Affects one's ability to express life force which resides in the Heart through articulation or through vision

- Invigorates a person to experience passion and manifest it

- Helps correct qi (body–mind–spirit) to rectify feelings of shame or guilt that are carried in this particular vessel so a person can shed habitual tendency of guilt

KIDNEY 8

- Regulates Chong Mai and Ren Mai

- Benefits the uterus, regulates menstruation; stops uterine bleeding; treats dysmenorrhea and amenorrhea

- Releases deficiency heat from Kidneys (menopausal hot flashes and night sweats, inappropriate sweating in general, lumbar pain)

- In combination with other points, releases heat from blood

- Resolves dampness, resolves damp-heat in the lower jiao

- Strongly influences the pelvic cavity (addresses many fertility issues, shan disorder)

- Restores faith in the self

- Helps a person identify the self and personal needs in cases where they are disconnected from their own needs (environmental, relational, physical, etc.)

- Offers a gateway to understand what is possible and what is right for self; provides spiritual direction

KIDNEY 11

- Benefits and regulates the lower jiao (seminal emissions, impotence, exhaustion of five zang, enuresis, lin syndrome, painful genitals, vaginismus, shan disorder)

- Resolves dampness and clears heat

- Treats extreme/acute pelvic disorders such as prolapse or cancers in the pelvic cavity in both females and males (prostate, uterine, etc.)

- Can be used in combination: Yin Qiao Mai + Chong Mai + **KI11** for fertility; also supports the Stomach and resolves damp conditions

- Can be used with **KI13** for herpes

KIDNEY 12

- Tonifies Kidneys and astringes essence (pain of genitals, impotence, seminal emission, leukorrhea, uterine prolapse)

- Regulates the uterus and menstruation

- Clears heat

- Can be used in combination: Yin Qiao Mai + Chong Mai + **KI11** for fertility; when combined with **KI12**, helps individual to manifest self-expression

- Supports healing from trauma

KIDNEY 13

- Tonifies Kidneys and essence

- Benefits the uterus and regulates Chong Mai and Ren Mai (amenorrhea, dysmenorrhea, uterine bleeding, leukorrhea)

- Regulates lower jiao and two lower orifices

- Clears heat

- Treats infertility (use this point alone with Yin Qiao Mai three times consecutively and evaluate; can repeat later, pairing with Chong Mai and adding **KI11/12**)

- Supports healing from trauma

KIDNEY 14

- Regulates uterus and lower jiao (dysmenorrhea, uterine bleeding, leukorrhea, retention of lochia, seminal emission, diarrhea/constipation)

- Nourishes the essence and marrow

- Alleviates pain, shan disorder, malign blood

- Treats stasis of qi, blood, fluids, and phlegm; regulates fluids throughout the body (edema)

- Clears cold accumulation in uterus, infertility (cysts or other phlegm issues of ovaries or uterus)

- Supports healing from trauma

KIDNEY 15

- Regulates intestines and lower jiao (diarrhea/constipation, dysmenorrhea, lumbar pain)

- Nourishes Kidneys and yin—most commonly used in Yin Qiao Mai

- Supports healing from trauma

KIDNEY 16

- Regulates qi, alleviates pain

- Regulates and warms intestines (diarrhea/constipation, borborygmus, vomiting, leaky gut syndrome, lin syndrome)

- Treats epigastric distention, pain or cold, shan disorder

- Nourishes Kidneys and yin—most commonly used in Yin Qiao Mai

- Supports healing from trauma

- Strengthens vitality of entire system

KIDNEY 17

- Dispels accumulation and alleviates pain

- Harmonizes the Stomach (abdominal masses, intestinal pain with lack of appetite, diarrhea/constipation, vomiting)

- Regulates and supports Spleen (great for Earth constitutions)

- Can be used in combination with **KI11** to strongly support Stomach/Spleen dynamic

- Treats blood in cases of depression/resignation—boosts mood; this point can be used to manage difficult emotions that may arise in the context of eight extraordinary vessel treatments

- Treats kidney stones and gallstones

KIDNEY 18

- Regulates lower jiao, alleviates pain (dark urine)

- Regulates qi, moves blood stasis (malign blood in uterus, infertility)

- Treats damp conditions in the middle jiao

- Harmonizes the Stomach/Spleen with the Liver and addresses rebellious qi (digestive issues)

- Overcomes inability to concentrate, foggy mind

- Helps break down the barriers/obstacles an individual has created due to habitual tendencies (self-sabotage)

- Unlocks gates to allow person to step into their power and get out of their own way

- Soothes fear of one's own power/potential

KIDNEY 19

- Regulates qi; addresses rebellious qi to stop cough and wheezing

- Treats fullness and agitation below the Heart

- Disperses malign blood in uterus, treats infertility
- Treats damp conditions in the middle jiao
- Harmonizes the Stomach/Spleen with the Liver and addresses rebellious qi (digestive issues)
- Overcomes inability to concentrate, foggy mind
- Helps break down the barriers/obstacles an individual has created due to habitual tendencies (self-sabotage)
- Unlocks gates to allow person to step into their power and get out of their own way
- Soothes fear of one's own power/potential
- Can be used in combination with **KI20** to help person ease transition
- Treats blood-related Spleen issues

KIDNEY 20

- Harmonizes the Stomach/Spleen with the Liver and addresses rebellious qi (digestive issues)
- Unbinds the chest and transforms phlegm
- Overcomes inability to concentrate, foggy mind
- Prevents palpitations, epilepsy, sudden loss of voice, deviation of the mouth, inability to turn the neck, protrusion or swelling of the tongue
- Helps break down the barriers/obstacles an individual has created due to habitual tendencies (self-sabotage)
- Unlocks gates to allow person to step into their power and get out of their own way
- Soothes fear of one's own power/potential
- Removes gui
- Can be used in combination with **KI19** to help person ease transition

KIDNEY 21

- Fortifies the Spleen (loss of appetite)

- Harmonizes the Stomach/Spleen with the Liver and addresses rebellious qi (digestive issues); stops vomiting

- Benefits the chest and breasts (cough, coughing blood, breast abscess, breast milk not flowing), alleviates pain

- Overcomes inability to concentrate, foggy mind, poor memory

- Helps break down the barriers/obstacles an individual has created due to habitual tendencies (self-sabotage)

- Unlocks gates to allow person to step into their power and get out of their own way

- Soothes fear of one's own power/potential

- Removes gui

- Can be used in cases when patient may need a buffer to emotional turmoil that arises during treatment; treats emotional turmoil

Kidney 22–27 are less commonly used as Yin Qiao Mai trajectory points.

KIDNEY 22

- Unbinds the chest

- Subdues rebellious Lung and Stomach qi

- Provides a sense of stability and security while simultaneously broadening one's horizons

- Opens a person's eyes to what may be possible while supporting and anchoring them in the familiar

KIDNEY 23

- Unbinds the chest; stops cough

- Harmonizes the Stomach and subdues rebellious Lung and Stomach qi

- Benefits the breasts
- Provides clarity regarding one's uniqueness and value
- Supports the integration of one's sense of self

KIDNEY 24

- Unbinds the chest, descends Lung qi
- Subdues rebellious Lung and Stomach qi
- Benefits the breasts
- Smooths the flow of Liver qi
- Reignites the spirit in cases of depression
- Soothes deep fears and nightmares
- Clears out the cobwebs of resignation to make room for the wisdom and flow of life

KIDNEY 25

- Unbinds the chest, descends Lung qi
- Subdues rebellious Lung and Stomach qi
- Treats worry, anxiety, and insomnia, especially when the patient is very depleted
- Strengthens the will

KIDNEY 26

- Unbinds the chest and benefits the breasts
- Transforms phlegm and subdues rebellious Lung and Stomach qi
- Treats asthma; moves obstruction out of chest and throat (patient may constantly be attempting to clear their throat)
- Reminds the patient to appreciate and respect the beauty within self and others

- Supports someone who feels discouraged or is "going through the motions"

KIDNEY 27

- Unbinds the chest, descends Lung qi, and stops cough

- Transforms phlegm and alleviates cough and wheezing

- Harmonizes the Stomach and subdues rebellious qi; stops vomiting

- Treats asthma; moves obstruction out of chest and throat (patient may constantly be attempting to clear their throat)

- Treats burnout, exhaustion, and severe irritability

- Rejuvenates spirit and replenishes energy reserves

STOMACH 1

- Brightens the eyes and stops lacrimation

- Expels wind and clears heat

- Assists with judgment

- Assists in the movement of vision (physiologically, metaphorically)

- Supports the ability to see clearly what lies ahead and digest what is seen

- Opens structure so a person is able to receive, discern, and disseminate the information appropriately

- Is great for someone who has a difficult time with discernment, which can create boundary issues

STOMACH 2

- Brightens the eyes

- Expels wind and clears heat

- Assists with judgment

- Assists in the movement of vision (physiologically, metaphorically)

- Supports the ability to see clearly what lies ahead and digest what is seen

- Opens structure so a person is able to receive, discern, and disseminate the information appropriately

- Is great for someone who has a difficult time with discernment, which can create boundary issues

STOMACH 3

- Expels wind, dissipates swelling, and alleviates pain

- Assists in regulating temperature, treats allergies; coupled with Kidney points, helps with inappropriate sweating

- Assists with judgment

- Assists in the movement of vision (physiologically, metaphorically)

- Supports the ability to see clearly what lies ahead and digest what is seen

- Opens structure so a person is able to receive, discern, and disseminate the information appropriately

- Is great for someone who has a difficult time with discernment, which can create boundary issues

STOMACH 4

- Expels wind from the face; treats acne

- Activates the channel and alleviates pain

- Treats eating disorders, addresses metabolism problems (in cases of unhealthy relationship with food, to help the person lose weight by identifying the issue and understanding how to make changes and manifest that shift, use Yin Qiao Mai + **ST4**, **SP4**, **CV10**)

- Assists with judgment

- Assists in the movement of vision (physiologically, metaphorically)

- Supports the ability to see clearly what lies ahead and digest what is seen

- Opens structure so a person is able to receive, discern, and disseminate the information appropriately

- Is great for someone who has a difficult time with discernment, which can create boundary issues

STOMACH 9

- Regulates vertical movement of qi and blood through the neck and subdues rebellion

- Benefits the throat and neck

- Dissipates nodules, alleviates pain

- Treats conditions related to glands (thyroid, adrenals)

- Facilitates vision—big-picture perspective

STOMACH 12

- Subdues rebellious qi; descends Lung qi and clears heat from the chest

- Activates the channel and alleviates pain

- Treats conditions related to glands (thyroid, adrenals)

- Facilitates vision—big-picture perspective

BLADDER 1

- Brightens the eyes

- Expels wind and clears heat; stops itching

- Treats neurological issues; specifically stimulates the pituitary gland

- Facilitates vision—big-picture perspective

GALLBLADDER 20

- Expels exterior wind and extinguishes internal wind
- Subdues Liver yang
- Clears heat
- Benefits the head and clears the sense organs
- Nourishes marrow and clears the brain
- Activates the channel and alleviates pain
- Treats wind conditions, releases exterior conditions, relaxes rigidity in thinking or rigidity that manifests in the body (when the rigidity has manifested into physical symptoms of stiffness, pair Yin Qiao Mai with Yang Qiao Mai + **GB20** (disperse); if rigidity exists in the mind only, use Yin Qiao Mai along with **GB34**)

Possible Off-Trajectory Points

Spleen 4

Gallbladder 34

Conception Vessel 10

SPLEEN 4

- Tonifies the Spleen and harmonizes the middle jiao
- Regulates the intestines
- Stops bleeding and regulates menstruation
- Regulates qi and resolves dampness
- Calms the spirit and opens the mind's orifices
- Benefits the Heart and chest
- Regulates the Chong Mai

- Benefits the feet and toes

- Treats eating disorders, addresses metabolism problems (in cases of unhealthy relationship with food, to help the person lose weight by identifying the issue and understanding how to make changes and manifest that shift, use Yin Qiao Mai + **ST4**, **SP4**, **CV10**)

GALLBLADDER 34

- Benefits the sinews and joints

- Activates the channel and alleviates pain

- Spreads Liver qi and benefits the lateral costal region

- Clears Liver and Gallbladder damp-heat

- Harmonizes Shao Yang

- Treats wind conditions and releases exterior conditions

- Relaxes rigidity in thinking or rigidity that manifests in the body (when the rigidity has manifested into physical symptoms of stiffness, pair Yin Qiao Mai with Yang Qiao Mai + **GB20** (disperse); if rigidity exists in the mind only, use Yin Qiao Mai with **GB34**)

CONCEPTION VESSEL 10

- Harmonizes the Stomach and regulates qi

- Resolves food stagnation

- Treats eating disorders, addresses metabolism problems (in cases of unhealthy relationship with food, to help the person lose weight by identifying the issue and understanding how to make changes and manifest that shift, use Yin Qiao Mai + **ST4**, **SP4**, **CV10**)

YANG QIAO MAI

Master point: BL62

Couple point: SI3

Common trajectory points:

BL61, 59

GB29

SI10

LI15, 16

ST4, 3, 2, 1

GB20

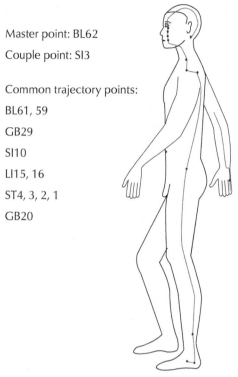

Figure 5.2 Yang Qiao Mai (Yang Heel Vessel)

Master Point: Bladder 62

Couple Point: Small Intestine 3

The Yang Qiao Mai binds the left and right sides together, traveling through the shoulders, with a zigzag pathway in the shoulder. There is debate concerning the exact trajectory, but there is a general consensus that the vessel traverses the shoulder area. From the shoulder area it courses through the neck and into the brain, assisting the functioning of the Yin Qiao Mai. Classical texts describe the shoulder, somewhere in the vicinity of Small Intestine 10, as the initial meeting point between the physical body and the environment. This point is on the Yang Qiao Mai, where we as humans meet the world in everyday life, which is why the burdens of the world are carried on our shoulders.

The Yang Qiao Mai is essentially where the individual "meets" their environment. The vessel travels along the side of the body and through the brain. This area is vulnerable to external pathogenic factors, but also environmental issues that lead to emotional stress, angst, or frustration. Generally speaking, the immediate environment impacts an individual as they experience life by influencing the Yang Qiao Mai level. The meeting between individual and environment begets perception; the individual observes the world around them, and those observations are translated in the mind. At this stage of discerning perception, the Yang Wei Mai comes into action, forming a connection between the Yang Qiao Mai and the Yang Wei Mai.

This immediate perception has an impact on the individual's view of the self. Additionally, the perception is quickly discerned and assimilated in both the Yin Wei Mai as well as the Yin Qiao Mai systems. These vessels work so interdependently that they are generally thought of as one unit or complete channel system. However, there are subtle differences. The Yin and Yang Wei Mai have more to do with internal perception and environmental impacts at the heart/spirit level, whereas the Yin and Yang Qiao Mai have more to do with external perception and environmental impacts at the body/mind level.

When a patient complains of chronic shoulder pain without injury or surgery, or that is otherwise inexplicable, there is an emotional etiology. Life's burdens are stored either in the Wei Mai or Qiao Mai. This is a good example of how the Qiao Mai and Wei Mai share the load of life's burdens. And because the Qiao Mai travel deep in the brain, they can be used successfully in treating wind conditions (e.g., Parkinson's disease, seizures, epilepsy, and other neurological disorders).

Pathology of the Yin or Yang Qiao Mai is certain to affect both vessels. Again, because of their close working relationship it is difficult to discuss one without the other. The Qiao Mai is associated with that which brings fury, madness, agitation, and inertia, breaking down the communication between yin and yang. When the patient is overloaded, overwhelmed with their life course, the nervous system is overcharged and no more information or stimuli can be received or integrated, so spiritual evolution is halted.

Disharmony most strongly associated with the Yang Qiao Mai includes severe feelings of being overwhelmed by past events, in most cases secret or hidden past experiences leading to depression, restlessness, and nervous tension. The patient will describe the feeling of being haunted by a past experience, being unable to let "it" go, and being plagued by thoughts about the situation. Insomnia and other types of sleep disharmonies may also be present.

Because the vessel travels into the brain just like the Yin Qiao Mai, issues with gait (walking physically as well as metaphorically), pain in the legs, especially down the sides, and neuropathy are associated with this vessel. As with the Yang Qiao Mai, neurological conditions (wind disturbances) can be treated on the Yin Qiao Mai.

The Yang Qiao Mai is also indicated for treating patients who are in a constant state of excessive rebellion such as extremists and activists who have gone too far in the pursuit of their cause. In harmony, the Yang Qiao Mai allows us to speak up about our passions and views, and to be assertive in a healthy manner. Those who set out to change the world for the better have a healthy Yang Qiao Mai, but when the vessel is in disharmony, that Yang spirit that allows for an expansion of the mind becomes diseased and people can take their actions too far, beyond what is morally accepted (e.g., shooting rampages, acts of terrorism).

Trajectory Points

Bladder 1, 59, and 61

Gallbladder 20, 29, and 39

Small Intestine 10

Large Intestine 15 and 16

Stomach 1, 3, and 4

BLADDER 1

- Brightens the eye
- Expels wind and clears heat; stops itching
- Neurological issues, specifically stimulates the pituitary gland
- Facilitates vision—big-picture perspective

BLADDER 59

- Benefits the lumbar region and legs

- Activates the channel and alleviates pain

- Invigorates the Yang Qiao Mai

- Treats seizure, Bell's palsy, stroke

- Treats compromised autoimmune system (fibromyalgia, Wegener's disease, Wilson's disease, leaky gut, chronic fatigue, lupus, Lyme disease)

- Pair Yin Qiao Mai with Yang Qiao Mai for immune issues; combine this point with **LI4** to release toxicity

- Creates movement forward spiritually in context of patient's newly found vision

BLADDER 61

- Relaxes the sinews, activates the channel, and alleviates pain (especially low back and leg pain)

- Eliminates damp-heat

- Treats wei qi issues

- This point is the body's personal assistant, similar to the relationship between the Lung and Heart (the Lung ministers the Heart), and it will serve the person in whatever way is needed— condensed essence of everything the Bladder channel has to offer (head to toe)

- Supports vision and taking action; creates fluid facilitation of the task at hand

GALLBLADDER 20

- Expels exterior wind and extinguishes internal wind

- Subdues Liver yang

- Clears heat

- Benefits the head and clears the sense organs

- Nourishes marrow and clears the brain

- Activates the channel and alleviates pain

- Treats wind conditions, releases exterior conditions, relaxes rigidity in thinking or rigidity that manifests in the body (when the rigidity has manifested into physical symptoms of stiffness, pair Yin Qiao Mai with Yang Qiao Mai + **GB20** (disperse); if rigidity exists in the mind only, use Yin Qiao Mai along with **GB34**)

GALLBLADDER 29

- Activates the channel and alleviates pain

- Benefits the hip joint; treats issues with the hips/gait/posture

- Is mostly used for physical symptoms such as back pain; add to point combination for physical manifestation of rigidity (Pair Yin Qiao Mai with Yang Qiao Mai + **GB20** + **GB29**)

- Brings fluidity to metaphoric movement through life as well

- Is not commonly used alone

- Treats damp-heat in the lower jiao

GALLBLADDER 39

- Regulates the Gall Bladder channel

- Extinguishes Liver Wind

- Clears Heat

- Helps to strengthen the bones

- Transforms Damp-Heat

- Benefits the ears

- Helps to drain excess qi from the upper part of the body

- In conjunction with the Liver channel, helps to facilitate flow of qi in the lower limbs

SMALL INTESTINE 10

- Moves blood and qi through shoulder girdle; benefits the shoulder
- Activates the channel and alleviates pain
- Is the place where we meet the world; helps in sorting out who is safe/appropriate socially; helps in discerning whether to stay or go with regard to interpersonal relationships
- Treats heat in the Heart

LARGE INTESTINE 15

- Dispels wind-damp, alleviates pain, and benefits the shoulder joint
- Eliminates wind and regulates qi and blood
- Regulates qi, resolves phlegm, and dissipates nodules
- Treats bowel symptoms and vomiting

LARGE INTESTINE 16

- Activates the channel, alleviates pain, and benefits the shoulder joint
- Regulates qi and blood and dissipates nodules
- Treats bowel symptoms and vomiting
- Pair with **GB20** for wind conditions

STOMACH 1

- Brightens the eyes and stops lacrimation
- Expels wind and clears heat
- Assists with judgment
- Assists in the movement of vision (physiologically, metaphorically)
- Supports the ability to see clearly what lies ahead and digest what is seen

- Opens structure so a person is able to receive, discern, and disseminate the information appropriately

- Is great for someone who has a difficult time with discernment, which can create boundary issues

STOMACH 3

- Expels wind, dissipates swelling, and alleviates pain

- Assists in regulating temperature, treats allergies; coupled with Kidney points, helps with inappropriate sweating

- Assists with judgment

- Assists in the movement of vision (physiologically, metaphorically)

- Supports the ability to see clearly what lies ahead and digest what is seen

- Opens structure so a person is able to receive, discern, and disseminate the information appropriately

- Is great for someone who has a difficult time with discernment, which can create boundary issues

STOMACH 4

- Expels wind from the face; treats acne

- Activates the channel and alleviates pain

- Treats eating disorders, addresses metabolism problems (in cases of unhealthy relationship with food, to help the person lose weight by identifying the issue and understanding how to make changes and manifest that shift, use Yin Qiao Mai + **ST4, SP4, CV10**)

- Assists with judgment

- Assists in the movement of vision (physiologically, metaphorically)

- Supports the ability to see clearly what lies ahead and digest what is seen

- Opens structure so a person is able to receive, discern, and disseminate the information appropriately

- Is great for someone who has a difficult time with discernment, which can create boundary issues

Possible Off-Trajectory Points

Spleen 4

Gallbladder 34 and 39

Conception Vessel 10

SPLEEN 4

- Tonifies the Spleen and harmonizes the middle jiao

- Regulates the intestines

- Stops bleeding and regulates menstruation

- Regulates qi and resolves dampness

- Calms the spirit and opens the mind's orifices

- Benefits the Heart and chest

- Regulates the Chong Mai

- Benefits the feet and toes

- Treats eating disorders, addresses metabolism problems (in cases of unhealthy relationship with food, to help the person lose weight by identifying the issue and understanding how to make changes and manifest that shift, use Yin Qiao Mai + **ST4**, **SP4**, **CV10**)

GALLBLADDER 34

- Benefits the sinews and joints

- Activates the channel and alleviates pain

- Spreads Liver qi and benefits the lateral costal region

- Clears Liver and Gallbladder damp-heat

- Harmonizes Shao Yang

- Treats wind conditions and releases exterior conditions

- Relaxes rigidity in thinking or rigidity that manifests in the body (when the rigidity has manifested into physical symptoms of stiffness, pair Yin Qiao Mai with Yang Qiao Mai + **GB20** (disperse); if rigidity exists in the mind only, use Yin Qiao Mai with **GB34**)

GALLBLADDER 39

- Benefits the sinews, bones, and marrow

- Benefits the neck

- Expels wind, dispels wind-damp

- Clears Gallbladder fire and subdues Liver yang

- Activates the channel and alleviates pain (treats low back pain)

- Treats rigidity in the pelvic cavity or lower extremities

- Loosens stiffness on the mental/physical level

- Treats autoimmune issues (great for treating multiple sclerosis)

- Pairs well with **GB29**

CONCEPTION VESSEL 10

- Harmonizes the Stomach and regulates qi

- Resolves food stagnation

- Treats eating disorders, addresses metabolism problems (in cases of unhealthy relationship with food, to help the person lose weight by identifying the issue and understanding how to make changes and manifest that shift, use Yin Qiao Mai + **ST4, SP4, CV10**)

QIAO MAI AND WEI MAI, IN REVIEW

To review, it is accepted practice to pair Yin Qiao Mai with Yin Wei Mai, and Yang Qiao Mai with Yang Wei Mai, but one would not normally pair Yin Qiao Mai with Yang Wei Mai or Yin Wei Mai with Yang Qiao Mai. Ideally, the pairings would be one of the following:

- Yin and Yang Qiao Mai
- Yin and Yang Wei Mai
- Yin Qiao Mai and Yin Wei Mai
- Yang Qiao Mai and Yang Wei Mai

The Qiao Mai and Wei Mai are continuously addressing the yin and yang energies. These four vessels can be viewed as holders of all that is yin and all that is yang. In fact, many practitioners focus exclusively on the Qiao Mai and Wei Mai in their treatment strategies with patients, consistently and methodically moving among the Qiao Mai, the Wei Mai, and the twelve primary meridians.

The Yin Wei Mai allows one to speak from their heart, to dance with the ups and downs of life. However, the functions of the Yin Wei Mai rely on the health and vitality of its counterpart, the Yin Qiao Mai. Harmony in both is needed in order for the person to be able to dance with life fully, appropriately, and with vitality. Because humans are highly intelligent and intricate systems of multiple energetic channels, the relationship between the Qiao Mai and Wei Mai can become complicated.

Subtle trajectories of these vessels intersect with the Chong Mai and some practitioners suggests this junction occurs at the sacral chakra. The connection with the Chong Mai, in the middle of the genital region, is the place where there is an opening for a higher spiritual connection. This helps explain why in most meditation practices the person sits in a particular posture that allows for an opening within the Central Channel (Chong Mai). The "essential air and fluids" are opened from the core of the person toward and through the crown to support the potential for the person to experience a spiritual ascent. Chapter 13 includes more detail about the essential air and fluids: what they are and why they are important in the context of the eight extraordinary vessels.

The Yang Wei Mai is associated with the future, but only in the context of a person who is speculating about the future (because they have not actually lived it) and projecting a picture on the future. In health, this vessel generates optimism and healthy planning without becoming obsessive or rigid.

YIN AND YANG WEI MAI

The Yin and Yang Wei Mai are generally paired together. Li Shi Zhen asserts that the close relationship between these vessels indicates that the practitioner should view them as inseparable. They are always in communication with one another (see Figure 5.3). The Yin Wei Mai contains the internal workings of the person, and the Yang Wei Mai is the person's external interface, where the individual meets their immediate environment. The environment, in turn, impacts the physical structure of their body.

To visualize how these vessels work, imagine a group of soldiers marching through a wooded area. They are in a specific file pattern based on enemy activity. In their particular environment, there is an immediate and heightened influence on their structure (i.e., their body, physically, emotionally, and spiritually). Their immediate environment is "meeting" them on the sides of their body, from shoulders to heels. The space between their bodies and the environment is so small it is virtually indistinguishable.

In this precise moment, the Yin Qiao Mai and the Yang Qiao Mai are hard at work; however, the Yin Wei Mai is also being impacted. The constant heightened awareness taxes the Yin Wei Mai because every detail of the intensely stressful situation is being recorded in memory and stored in the tissue and molecular makeup of the body.

The Yin Wei Mei and the Yang Wei Mei are known as the recorders of our experiences, the autobiographies of our lives. When there is over-collection of data, the vessels become too full and, consequently, an excess condition begins to develop. This helps explain why we want to work on the Yin Wei Mai prior to the Chong Mai or Dai Mai when it comes to reducing accumulation. The Yin Wei Mai tongue expression can be almost identical to the Chong Mai tongue presentation. This will be discussed more thoroughly in the treatment planning section.

These vessels are not gender specific, meaning they function the same regardless of gender. Other vessels can present issues differently with respect to gender, but this is not so when it comes to the Qiao Mai and Wei Mai.

The Wei Mai are often described as the tapestry of our lives, the complete journey of life from birth to death. The tapestry can become very tight at times and almost unravel at other times. When a person possesses healthy Wei Mai, they can dance with life regardless of the ups and downs, births and deaths, through joy and sadness. On the other hand, when the

Wei Mai are not vital and healthy, a person has a difficult time with coping, and can literally become stuck and unable to fully move forward in life.

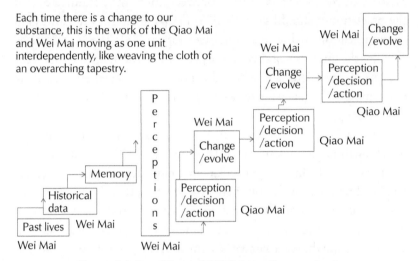

Each time there is a change to our substance, this is the work of the Qiao Mai and Wei Mai moving as one unit interdependently, like weaving the cloth of an overarching tapestry.

Figure 5.3 Qiao Mai and Wei Mai in Communication

YIN WEI MAI

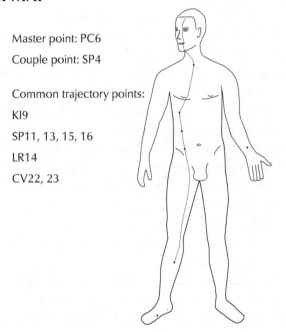

Master point: PC6

Couple point: SP4

Common trajectory points:

KI9

SP11, 13, 15, 16

LR14

CV22, 23

Figures 5.4a Yin Wei Mai (Yin Linking Vessel)—Male

Master point: PC6

Couple point: SP4

Common trajectory points:

KI9

SP11, 13, 15, 16

LR14

CV22, 23

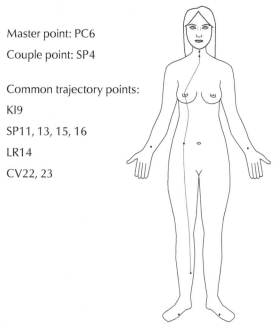

Figure 5.4b Yin Wei Mai (Yin Linking Vessel)—Female

Master Point: Pericardium 6

Couple Point: Spleen 4

The Yin Wei Mai binds the interior and exterior of the body, connecting all yin channels. When there is an over-collection in the Yin Wei Mai, it ultimately impacts all of the yin organ officials. The person will feel imbalanced and multiple symptoms will be present. The accumulation will be expressed primarily based upon the constitutional nature of the person. In other words, accumulation in the Yin Wei Mai will manifest in the zang organ that corresponds to the patient's constitutional factor (CF) as determined by five element theory (e.g., accumulation in the Heart of a Fire CF, Spleen of an Earth CF). However, in broad general expressions, a more classic sign and symptom of excess in the Yin Wei Mai will be expressed in the Heart and Pericardium, manifesting primarily in the emotional body, as apprehension, a lack of trust, feeling emotionally torn or inappropriately emotional, pensive, and obsessive. Phobias and anxiety may be experienced, and in extreme cases, paranoia. At this level, the person will not be able to go out of the house without certain conditions being met. The most common example is known as post-traumatic stress disorder (PTSD). Many military members who have been in combat or combat-like situations experience these symptoms as a result of accumulation in the Yin Wei Mai.

The Yin Wei Mai is the gate to the inner self. If closed, it makes internal alchemy difficult, if not impossible, to achieve. Traumas, heartbreaks, and high stress are the cause for accumulation in the Heart. When the accumulation hits individual thresholds, the gate closes and thus the person shuts themselves off from the ability to love unconditionally. In some cases, it becomes difficult for the person to develop appropriate interpersonal relationships. Can the person still love despite multiple broken-heart situations? If the gate is closed, and is not able to open, the spirit of the person begins to die. The Pericardium rules the gate to the Heart, and this is why Pericardium 6 is used as the MP to help activate the channel. The couple point is used for two main reasons: for its deep trajectory in the body and association with the Heart, and for its grounding mechanism. Without using both the master point and the couple point, the channel is not fully activated; therefore both points are required to fully activate the channel.

In terms of treatment protocols, it is best to start treating a patient on the Qiao Mai before moving to the Wei Mai. However, if the practitioner has adequately assessed that the gate to the patient's inner self is closed, it may prove useful to treat this vessel first in order to open the gate. It is not uncommon to treat the Yin Wei Mai as many as five times in order to fully open the gate. The more trauma the person has endured and/or the more profound *their perception* of that trauma, the more tightly closed the gate is and the more closed off the person becomes to the world. As with any of the eight extraordinary vessels, it is important for the patient to have a supportive environment as they begin to process and clear the pathology that rests in these deeper vessels.

Physical symptoms may be expressed with heart pain, palpitations, restlessness, affected shen, low back pain, depression/fear, dizziness, and possibly fainting. There are essentially nine major types of emotional pain affecting the Heart that contribute to the gate being closed full-time, resulting in pathology. The Nine Heart Pains are emotional distress regarding money, prosperity, health, career, vocation, relationships, children and/or creativity or lack thereof, adventure, and cultivation of a sense of home. Stresses experienced in these nine domains deplete the spirit of the Heart and lead to pathology in the Yin Wei Mai.

Because the Wei Mai are the recorders of our lives, memories are stored in these vessels and can show up as pathological accumulations in any of the yin officials: Heart, Spleen, Lung, Kidney, or Liver. The state of excess in the Spleen is expressed as significant qi or blood stagnation, in the Lung as panting, in the Kidney as panic attacks, in the Liver as fatty deposits, and in the Heart as hidden beam—an accumulation that arises from the umbilicus area upward to just under the Heart, afflicting the Heart and Pericardium. The most common symptom is spitting blood, accompanied with vexation. A patient can have more than one type of accumulation. The manifestations listed can at first glance present on the tongue as a Chong Mai accumulation. It is best for the practitioner not to jump to this conclusion too quickly.

A potential treatment protocol typically progresses from the Qiao Mai, to the Wei Mai, and then to the four primaries. It is helpful to have a "target" vessel and work patiently toward that target vessel. To address any of the accumulations, it can prove beneficial to treat the Chong Mai; however, unless there is a strong and convincing reason to treat the Chong Mai first, it would best to start with the Yin Wei Mai to address the gate closure condition. Additionally, the Yin Wei Mai is regarded as the transitional vessel from the Qiao Mai and Wei Mai to the four primaries (Chong Mai, Ren Mai, Du Mai, and Dai Mai). Therefore, it is more prudent to start with the Yin Wei Mai, especially in cases of accumulation and/or Pericardium gate closure.

It is true that phlegm (in general terms), tumors, fibroids, prolapsed organs (specifically bladder), and muscle atrophy in the lower limbs are more reflective of accumulation in the Dai Mai. However, because the Dai Mai binds all the vessels, it is potentially quite dangerous to open this vessel first. When the Dai Mai is opened prematurely, it is described as opening Pandora's box. It is more beneficial to design a treatment strategy that allows for a more thoughtful progression of healing for the patient, clearing from the outside inward. This is done by treating the Qiao Mai and Wei Mai prior to treating the primaries of the eight extraordinary vessels. When the Qiao Mai and Wei Mai have been properly treated, the individual experiences a solid, grounded, and healthy structure internally as well as externally, allowing a safe and grounded place to begin the deeper work of the Chong Mai, Ren Mai, Du Mai, and Dai Mai.

It is important for the Yin Wei Mai to be healthy because it is an instrumental vessel for the person to fulfill their life's work in the present life. In health, the Yin Wei Mai clears the path for the person's fulfillment of their destiny. Without a healthy Yin Wei Mai, the person will continue to struggle to achieve their highest potential.

Trauma can take many different forms. Gate closures can also result from living inauthentically. It is important we all walk our paths genuinely and compassionately. A healthy Yin Wei Mai not only allows for the individual to succeed but allows them to rejoice for others.

Trajectory Points

Kidney 9

Spleen 13, 15, and 16

Liver 14

Conception Vessel 22 and 23

KIDNEY 9

- Clears the Heart and transforms phlegm; opens the chest
- Calms the spirit and opens the mind's orifices
- Tonifies Kidney yin
- Regulates the Yin Wei Mai
- Regulates qi and alleviates pain
- Helps the person break free from the cycle of obsessiveness about the past (trauma, grief), helps to alleviate anxiety, with moxa on the needle

SPLEEN 13

- Regulates qi and alleviates pain
- Helps with assimilation in the midst of chaos experienced in life

- Moves stagnation of damp accumulation due to obsessiveness; disperses accumulations

SPLEEN 15

- Tonifies the Spleen and limbs

- Regulates qi and benefits the intestines

- Resolves dampness

SPLEEN 16

- Regulates the intestines (treats diarrhea, supports physical and emotional digestion)

- Quintessential point for treating sorrow in the context of the Yin Wei Mai; helps assuage remorse with a sense of a person's own contribution to current circumstances

LIVER 14

- Spreads and regulates Liver qi

- Invigorates blood and disperses masses

- Harmonizes the Liver and Stomach

- Offers a broader sense of perception and understanding of the current moment

CONCEPTION VESSEL 22

- Descends rebellious Lung qi and alleviates cough and wheezing

- Benefits the throat and voice

- Addresses plum pit qi and resolves phlegm

- Supports the breath and clarifies the voice

- Treats heartbreak; helps the person let go; calms the shen

- Restores all yin channels

- Needles in this point are not to be retained; rather, quickly tonified

CONCEPTION VESSEL 23

- Benefits the tongue and speech

- Descends rebellious qi and alleviates cough

- Addresses plum pit qi and other obstructions such as phlegm

- Supports the breath and clarifies the voice

- Treats heartbreak; helps the person let go; calms the shen

- Restores all yin channels

- Needles in this point are not to be retained; rather, quickly tonified

Possible Off-Trajectory Points

Spleen 8

Liver 9

SPLEEN 8

Spleen 8 is the blood of the Earth; it motivates, tills, and supports the Spleen meridian, so it is useful in addressing issues of fertility, blood disorders, and most types of cancer. From a spiritual perspective, it provides a level of grounding and centering like no other point on the trajectory and nourishes the spirit of the blood as it makes it way throughout the kingdom of an individual. When used in the context of the Yin Wei Mai, it is instrumental in mending a broken heart from the deepest levels to the exterior; from the yuan level to the wei level, it heals from the inside out. Its greatest strength is proven when combined with Spleen 15 in the context of the Yin Wei Mai, and it provides healing and support to the individual in most emotional distresses, especially in the recovery of a broken spirit whether the cause originated from a tragic disease, heartbreak, or trauma.

When the Spleen becomes sluggish or distressed, often disharmony manifests as menstrual issues and any irregular patterns in the function of a woman's uterus, including infertility, as well as fluid and fatty build-up in the body. It is also uniquely poised to assist with Kidney qi.

From a mental perspective, it can add flexibility to a rigid or narrow-minded individual whose stubborn nature is an obstacle to their emotional growth and development. It tills the hardened and barren Earth, nourishing and increasing the flow of blood and qi, and therefore offers a different perspective and experience of receiving sustenance.

In summary, it supports issues of the lower jiao: infertility, urinary issues, pelvic floor prolapses, and fatty tissue or fluid build-up, as common examples. It plants new seeds for growing and vitality. It shakes up the Earth element, tills the soil, harmonizes the pulses, and brings a smile to an otherwise barren face.

LIVER 9

Much like Spleen 8, Liver 9 is instrumental in addressing issues of fertility, and lower jiao issues in general. Given that it is on the Liver meridian, it is useful for agitation, irritation, and wind conditions. Therefore, for a patient who exhibits conditions related to wind in the context of the Yin Wei Mai, this is an excellent choice. When the Heart and spirit become disheveled, disorganized, or distressed, wind can kick up in the system and cause tremors, irregular uterine bleeding, abdominal cramping, and cramping in general.

While Liver 9 is a great point for many physical ailments, it is just as useful for emotional and mental issues. It helps relieve emotional pain in the same manner as physical pain. It is a natural mood stabilizer and disperses anxiousness to eliminate it. It alleviates the physical and emotional effects one experiences from chronic health diseases, including responses to chemotherapy. Liver 9 addresses chronic and lingering emotional disturbances such as depression, anxiety, and associated fatigue and stamina deficiencies.

In terms of needle action, Spleen 8 can be thrusted and tonified in the context of the Yin Wei Mai treatment, whereas Liver 9 should either be gently tonified or inserted using an "even technique," to avoid further irritation. A gentle nudge usually gets the job done.

YANG WEI MAI

Master point: TB5

Couple point: GB41

Common trajectory points:

BL63

GB35, 29

SI10

TB15

GB21, 14, 13, 16, 17, 18, 19, 20

GV15, 16

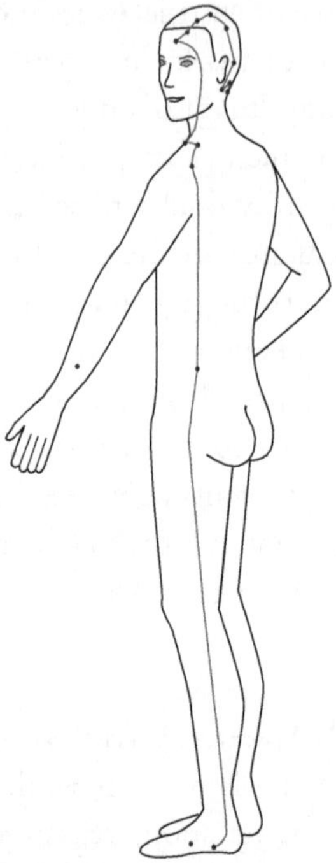

Figure 5.5 Yang Wei Mai (Yang Linking Vessel)

Master Point: Triple Burner/Heater 5

Couple Point: Gallbladder 41

The Yang Wei Mai is the recorder of the individual's autobiography in terms of action and major events in their life. It essentially dominates the exterior of the body. Whereas the Yang Qiao Mai is associated more with the structure of the body, and is where the individual meets the world, the Yang Wei Mai shares those responsibilities and is impacted by major life changes. Recall that the Qiao Mai bind the left and right sides of the body and the Wei Mai bind the interior and exterior of the body. This system of interior/exterior and sides of the body should be viewed as a unified channel system. The vessels work so interdependently with one another that it would be a grave oversight to view them as separate or isolated vessels.

The individual's level of optimism on a broad scale is housed in the Yang Wei Mai. This means that a healthy Yang Wei Mai leads to appropriate and healthy optimism. When there is pathology in the Yang Wei Mai, there is obsessiveness on a broad scale. This is seen most clearly when one is obsessive about one's life's work, career path, and the future. It is an inappropriate obsessiveness, not to be confused with ambition.

The Gallbladder–Heart axis, also known as the Liver–Heart axis (used somewhat interchangeably) is a spiritual conception which allows a person to live life from the Heart, aware of a broad perspective in service to one's destiny. This axis is indirectly impacted during Yang Wei Mai treatments. Treating the Yang Wei Mai essentially provides patients the opportunity for renewal and allows them to access optimism.

Classical physical symptoms of Yang Wei Mai pathology include chills, fever, aversion to cold or high fevers, difficulty regulating body temperature, forgetfulness, confusion, and perhaps even a lack of self-control. From an emotional point of view, pathology in this vessel will be expressed as an inability to make decisions or to let go of certain life events or situations, a lack of trust, and inaction on one's part to resolve conflict (i.e., a general lack of taking responsibility).

A healthy Yang Wei Mai will empower a person to gain focus, trust others, and engage in appropriate intimate interpersonal relationships. The Liver official plays a role in the Yang Wei's domain of cultivating vision and taking action in proportion to the vision. It provokes a transformational path for the individual. Therefore, the Liver channel has not only physical or emotional implications but also a deep and spiritual connection within the Qiao Mai/Wei Mai dynamic.

Because the Yang Wei Mai connects all the yang officials in the body, it is important to remember that many pathogenic factors and negative emotions are best released through the yang channel systems. Accordingly, the Yang Wei Mai plays an important role in releasing the past, resolving toxicity, and clearing pathogens. It does so through a myriad of physical avenues: fever/chills and sweat, bowel movements, urination, vertex headaches, and via the orifices.

Energetically, the Yang Wei Mai regulates old habits and patterns, and the release of these established modes of behavior that prevent the individual from evolving. The Yang Wei Mai assists the individual in moving forward in life.

It is important to note that the Yang Wei Mai is the last stage of defense before the body is penetrated by an invading pathogen; this vessel can therefore be used to treat terminal illness such as cancer or AIDS.

The intention in treating the Wei Mai is to give the patient a sense of perspective about not only their current life but the succession of their lives, like pearls along a string, and the interconnectedness of our lives from one to the next. This allows the person to become more focused on the present life with intention. It gives the patient the opportunity to renew their expectations with their life. Healthy Wei Mai allow individuals to dance more freely within the context of a larger framework.

To review, when treating a patient on the Qiao Mai and/or Wei Mai, there is no need to work in tandem with other theories such as eight principles or five elements. The practitioner would treat each vessel three times, using trajectory points as necessary. Again, pairing is an acceptable practice; however, once the practitioner begins treating on the four primary vessels (Chong Mai, Ren Mai, Du Mai, and Dai Mai), the patient would benefit from a break between each of the primary vessels for a period of time in which the practitioner would apply other treatment modalities. For example, the practitioner would treat on the Chong Mai a series of three times, using trajectory points if necessary, and once the series of three is completed, the practitioner would return to an eight principle or five element approach for a few treatments prior to moving on to the Ren Mai or Du Mai. The purpose behind this method of treating is to give the patient time to respond to the deeper vessel treatments. It fosters a more compassionate process.

> The Wei and the Qiao are best understood as two functional pairs... (Li Shi Zhen, cited in Chase and Shima, 2010, p.30)

Essentially, Li believed that the Wei Mai and the Qiao Mai can address any issue that comes into the treatment room and even promote internal alchemy and spiritual development. Further, the practitioner can treat these vessels alone or prior to the four primaries of the extraordinary vessels. Either way, there are plenty of opportunities for deep work.

Trajectory Points

Bladder 63

Gallbladder 13–21, 29, and 35

Large Intestine 14

Triple Burner 13–15

Small Intestine 10

BLADDER 63

- Pacifies wind

- Moderates acute conditions

- Relaxes the sinews

- Activates the channel and alleviates pain

- Supportive in wei qi issues

- Soothes fright/fear, provides sense of calm in the midst of chaos one perceives

- Helps resolve an issue from the past that is creating an obstacle in the current circumstances

- Can be used with **GB35**

GALLBLADDER 13

- Calms the spirit

- Subdues Liver yang

- Extinguishes wind, resolves phlegm, and treats epilepsy

- Gathers essence to the head; clears the brain

GALLBLADDER 14

- Subdues Liver yang

- Extinguishes interior wind, benefits the head, and alleviates pain

- Brightens the eyes

GALLBLADDER 15

- Subdues Liver yang

- Extinguishes interior wind

- Benefits the head and alleviates pain
- Benefits the nose and eyes
- Calms the spirit
- Can be combined with **GB16** to help a person express themselves
- Calms the shen, especially during difficult times

GALLBLADDER 16

- Benefits the eyes
- Eliminates wind and alleviates pain
- Can be combined with **GB15** to help one express oneself
- Calms the shen, especially during difficult times

GALLBLADDER 17

- Subdues Liver yang
- Resolves phlegm and opens the mind's orifices
- Benefits the head and alleviates pain
- Pacifies the Stomach

GALLBLADDER 18

- Subdues Liver yang
- Calms the spirit and opens the mind's orifices
- Benefits the head and alleviates pain
- Benefits the nose and descends Lung qi
- Can be combined with **GB19** to support a person's will to live and carry on; helps person remember to be present for other people, reminds one of responsibilities
- Treats indecision
- Assists the Spleen with head issues (sinus symptoms, nosebleeds, memory loss, neck issues, etc.)

GALLBLADDER 19

- Subdues Liver yang

- Clears Gallbladder channel heat

- Calms the spirit

- Benefits the head and alleviates pain

- Pacifies wind and clears the sense organs

- Can be combined with **GB18** to support a person's will to live and carry on; helps person remember to be present for other people, reminds one of responsibilities

- Treats indecision

- Assists the Spleen with head issues (sinus symptoms, nosebleeds, memory loss, neck issues, etc.)

GALLBLADDER 20

- Expels exterior wind and extinguishes internal wind

- Subdues Liver yang

- Clears heat

- Benefits the head and clears the sense organs

- Nourishes marrow and clears the brain

- Activates the channel and alleviates pain

- Treats wind conditions, releases exterior conditions, relaxes rigidity in thinking or rigidity that manifests in the body

GALLBLADDER 21

- Relaxes the sinews

- Regulates qi, activates the channel, and alleviates pain

- Transforms phlegm and resolves nodules

- Benefits the breasts, expedites delivery (by descending qi), and promotes lactation

- Descends Lung qi

GALLBLADDER 29

- Activates the channel and alleviates pain
- Benefits the hip joint
- Is mostly used for physical symptoms such as back pain or physical rigidity
- Treats issues with the hips/gait/posture; loosens hips
- Treats damp-heat in the lower jiao
- Brings fluidity to metaphoric movement through life as well
- Is not commonly used alone

GALLBLADDER 35

- Activates the channel and alleviates pain
- Regulates Gallbladder qi and calms the spirit
- Helps a person who feels panicked about life's transitions

LARGE INTESTINE 14

- Activates the channel and alleviates pain
- Regulates qi and resolves phlegm nodules
- Brightens the eyes

TRIPLE BURNER 13

- Regulates qi and transforms phlegm nodules
- Activates the channel and alleviates pain

TRIPLE BURNER 14

- Dispels wind-damp
- Alleviates pain and benefits the shoulder joint

TRIPLE BURNER 15

- Dispels wind-damp

- Activates the channel and alleviates pain

- Unbinds the chest and regulates qi

- Clears heat

SMALL INTESTINE 10

- Moves blood and qi through shoulder girdle; benefits the shoulder

- Activates the channel and alleviates pain

- Is the place where we meet the world; helps in sorting out who is safe/appropriate socially; helps in discerning whether to stay or go with regard to interpersonal relationships

- Treats heat in the Heart

Possible Off-Trajectory Points

Spleen 19–21

Gallbladder 29, 30, 38

Spleen 19, 20, and 21 offer similar patterns of relief in cases of thoracic fullness, upper jiao fullness, upper respiratory issues including asthma and bronchitis, and general aches and pains. Consider the spirit of each point to differentiate and select one of these while treating in the context of the Yang Wei Mai.

SPLEEN 19
Spleen 19 is generally used more for the physical benefits as opposed to emotional, mental, or spiritual. It helps to open the chest cavity for ease of breath, and to descend the qi when it is struggling to properly move through the upper jiao. It is a great point to add if the patient is currently coughing or wheezing or has a cold or virus that is impacting breath.

SPLEEN 20
Spleen 20 is a better point for the physical if the pulmonary issues are also

impacting the back, such as upper back discomfort or pain, or specific pain in the breast. Spleen 19 is more general while Spleen 20 is more specific in terms of signs and symptoms. One way to determine whether to add Spleen 19 or Spleen 20 (and you can always elect to do both) is if the patient is specifically complaining of difficulty breathing with back pain (usually in the flank area of the back) which is often because of chronic coughing. If the patient is not specifically complaining of back discomfort or chronic cough, Spleen 19 is a great point.

SPLEEN 21

The most beautiful quality of Spleen 21 is that it brings harmony to the entire meridian system, whether the intention is to bring harmony on a physical, emotional, or spiritual level. If the intent is to tend to the patient on the physical level, Spleen 19 and 20 are both excellent points; however, if the intent is to tend to the patient on a spiritual level, Spleen 21 is a far more appropriate point.

While it obviously offers benefit in opening the chest, allowing for deep breath, assisting with pain in the upper jiao, and regulating qi and blood, Spleen 21 is a great point to add for depression, lethargy, low motivation, and disorganization. Often when people experience a traumatic event, and these types of signs and symptoms occur (including common cold symptoms), they can become disheveled, disorganized, scattered, with feelings of being overwhelmed. In these cases, Spleen 21 is the better choice. It is the junction point of all junction points, especially when used in the context of an extraordinary vessel treatment. It is not only a grounding point but a nourishing point, and offers extraordinary support. It empowers the individual to feel solid within themselves, well, and connected.

GALLBLADDER 29 (AND 30)

While these points are mostly used for physical pain and discomfort, they do lend themselves to treating spiritual imbalances as well. Pain or discomfort originating from a previous life can be lodged in the hips, and in fact this is common. Certainly, one can have trauma or injury from the present life, but if the person continues to experience pain or discomfort in the hip area after multiple attempts with other treatment approaches, a Yang Wei Mai treatment using both GB29 and GB30 can be helpful in resolving the past-life karma lodged in the hip. In this instance, applying a thrusting needle action to the points is appropriate, followed by dispersing action.

Hypothetically, a person has been treated for chronic hip pain and after multiple attempts using various theories, including the eight extraordinary vessels, the patient continues to experience hip pain. Perhaps the pain occurs less frequently or less intensely, but still causes discomfort from time to time or with certain activities. Revisiting the Yang Wei Mai and including GB29 and GB30 allows the past-life trauma enough time to emerge from the cellular level and exit the tissues. In this case, it is recommended to apply a thrusting action (for trajectory points only, not for the MP or CP) initially, followed by dispersing and retaining all needles for as long as 40 minutes. This treatment may need to be repeated multiple times, depending on the nature of the pain and the length of time the patient has lived with the issue. The practitioner needs to take into account any structural issues that may be present and represented on imaging. For example, if the patient is experiencing bone on bone or other types of structural issues, acupuncture can help with releasing heat (inflammation) and assist the healing process, but the patient may still need some type of surgery to remedy the structural issue.

Some common themes that may indicate the need for pairing these points include difficulty with direction, follow through, or moving forward with projects, personal or professional or both. If after several treatments and perhaps even other modalities (e.g., physical therapy, chiropractic work, etc.) the hip pain continues, the indecisiveness gets worse, and other symptoms begin to emerge (eye issues and connective tissue problems are some common adjunct problems), these points are recommended.

From an emotional standpoint, the patient experiences weariness with an underlying sadness (teary or close to tears at any moment—they may cry in private), and their thinking becomes more rigid. In fact, the rigidity can manifest both mentally and physically. People who appear stiff physically often have rigid mindsets as well. In some cases, this is described as "stubborn" or "unbending." They lose perspective, becoming overly reactionary and argumentative. Underneath, and not spoken of, lie fear, anxiousness, and restlessness. A patient may be able to describe the feelings, but not what is causing them. If the trauma is from a past-life situation, the person will not be able to identify a cause and will become more frustrated; or they may make something up in their mind regarding the origin, but will not know for sure or believe their own story.

It is difficult for humans to live in the unknown, especially when there is pain with an unknown origin.

GALLBLADDER 38

Gallbladder 38 is associated more closely with the mental experience, as opposed to the physical. While it shares a common theme with many Gallbladder points (e.g., tightness, rigidity, soreness, pain, vision problems, and so on), it is more about the perspective and emotions of the person. The patient will sigh a lot when speaking, have a more negative outlook on life, and seem to have no vision for the future. This is not to be confused with fatalistic thinking, which is associated with the Chong Mai. Rather, in this case there is more a depressive connotation in general, with pain either in the hips, connective tissue (anywhere in the body including fingers and toes), joints, migraines or headaches, low back pain, middle jiao discomfort, and signs of wind as well.

These patients need a ray of sunshine to enter their lives to get back on track, and that ray of sunshine could be a shift in perspective, not necessarily literal sunlight. They are in a rut or a hole and have lost their ability to navigate out of the rut. The light at the end of the tunnel, so to speak, has gone, but they have not yet lost hope—they just feel discouraged. Opening the Yang Wei Mai and adding in GB38 will shift their perspective, allowing them to see their future once again, make a plan, or decide to alter the course they are seeking. It gives them optimism and reassurance for the future.

THE FOUR PRIMARIES: CHONG MAI, REN MAI, DU MAI, AND DAI MAI

Treat these vessels using caution. The key to a successful treatment is grounding the patient by performing leg pulls, applying moxa to Conception Vessel 8, or tonifying Kidney 3. Ensuring the patient is grounded before initiating the treatment supports them to have a safe and positive experience during the activation of the extraordinary vessel(s).

Other important items to note include how well the patient sleeps; on the day of an extraordinary vessel treatment, it is important the patient is not overly exhausted. Chronic sleep deprivation could predispose a patient to a disruption in equilibrium in response to an extraordinary vessel treatment.

Ensuring the patient has eaten prior to treatment allows extra fuel for the treatment and improves the likelihood of treatment success. Last but certainly not least, is hydration. It is important to ensure the patient has consumed an adequate amount of water during the day prior to treatment.

These key ingredients set the patient up for a successful treatment and provide a safe environment for the treatment to take place.

CHONG MAI

Master Point: Spleen 4

Couple Point: Pericardium 6

The Chong Mai is the Central Channel of the body, and the body/mind originates from the Chong Mai. Mind stream refers to the continuously evolving string of pearls discussed earlier and could holistically equate to the soul, where consciousness is housed. As one is reborn into the next life, the mind stream, which carries the karma, goes from the bardo of death into the bardo of life, and the cycle starts again. At conception, the mind stream travels from one bardo to the next, giving rise to pre-natal and post-natal qi, looking for what is familiar. Based on the karmic conditions of the mind stream and while in the bardo of death, parents are selected, and life begins again. Also, at that point, in addition to the eight extraordinary vessels being quite active, the twelve primary meridians begin to take form. All phenomena come from the five elements. As the Chong Mai is activated at the moment a woman becomes pregnant, the eight extraordinary vessels and twelve primaries begin working together.

The Chong Mai is an expression of the person's relationship with the priorities of the mind stream—destiny. While karmic conditions set the stage, their destiny is not set in stone and can be altered at any moment in one's life based on choices, environment, and the winds of karma. The Chong Mai does, however, hold the patterns that shape the growth and development cycles of the individual. It contains the jing the individual will need and brings yuan qi in the form of yin and yang to the Ren Mai and Du Mai. The Chong Mai is responsible for the individual's ability to discern their true nature.

There are a total of five Chong Mai trajectories. They each use the same MP and CP; however, trajectory points are selected based on the intention of the practitioner, in terms of which part of the Chong Mai is being treated. Depending upon which trajectory within the Chong Mai is determined to be most beneficial for the patient, additional points are selected on that particular pathway. The primary trajectory of the Chong Mai is most commonly used with patients in activating the Chong Mai. However, it is important to note that different aspects of the Chong Mai can be activated based on the diagnostic evaluation.

The first and primary trajectory travels within the pelvic cavity and becomes active at the moment of conception. The Chong Mai has a direct relationship with what is referred to as the Kidney–Heart axis and supports the Pericardium and Spleen meridians. This vessel can be used to treat any condition within the pelvic cavity for both men and women. It can also be influential in treating syndromes related to blood deficiency. It is vital to treat this trajectory when working with fertility patients.

Advanced practitioners may elect to pair the Ren Mai and Chong Mai in specific cases of infertility with a history of failed pregnancies. After exhausting other treatment strategies in efforts to support fertility, these vessels may be treated together. When a patient becomes pregnant, regardless of the treatment approach leading up to this moment, it is strongly recommended to cease treatment of the extraordinary vessels and resume eight principle or five element treatment strategies to support the pregnancy.

Master point: SP4

Couple point: PC6

Common trajectory points:

ST30

KI11–21

CV23

GV1, 4

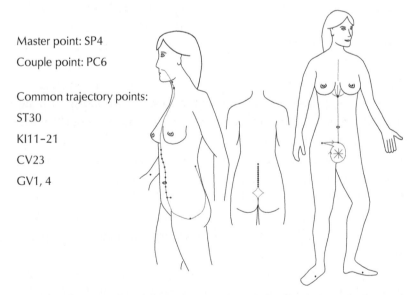

Figure 5.6 Chong Mai (Thrusting Vessel, Sea of Blood)—Primary Trajectory

Trajectory Points (Primary Trajectory)

Conception Vessel 2

Kidney 11–21

Stomach 30

Spleen 12

CONCEPTION VESSEL 2

- Benefits the Bladder and regulates urination
- Regulates lower jiao
- Warms and invigorates the Kidneys; consolidates the essence

KIDNEY 11

- Benefits and regulates the lower jiao (seminal emissions, impotence, exhaustion of five zang, enuresis, lin syndrome, painful genitals, vaginismus, shan disorder)
- Resolves dampness and clears heat
- Treats extreme/acute pelvic disorders such as prolapse or cancers in the pelvic cavity in both females and males (prostate, uterine, etc.)
- Can be used in combination: Yin Qiao Mai + Chong Mai + **KI11** for fertility; also supports the Stomach and resolves damp conditions
- Can be used with **KI13** for herpes

KIDNEY 12

- Tonifies Kidneys and astringes essence (painful genitals, impotence, seminal emission, leukorrhea, uterine prolapse)
- Regulates the uterus and menstruation
- Clears heat
- Can be used in combination: Yin Qiao Mai + Chong Mai + **KI11** for fertility; when combined with **KI12**, helps individual to manifest self-expression; supports healing from trauma

KIDNEY 13

- Tonifies Kidneys and essence
- Benefits the uterus and regulates Chong Mai and Ren Mai (amenorrhea, dysmenorrhea, uterine bleeding, leukorrhea)
- Regulates lower jiao and two lower orifices
- Clears heat
- Treats infertility (use this point alone with Yin Qiao Mai three times consecutively and evaluate; can repeat later pairing with Chong Mai and adding **KI11/12**)
- Supports healing from trauma

KIDNEY 14

- Regulates uterus and lower jiao (dysmenorrhea, uterine bleeding, leukorrhea, retention of lochia, seminal emission, diarrhea/ constipation)
- Nourishes the essence and marrow
- Alleviates pain, shan disorder, malign blood
- Treats stasis of qi, blood, fluids, and phlegm; regulates fluids throughout the body (edema)
- Clears cold accumulation in uterus, infertility (cysts or other phlegm issues of ovaries or uterus)
- Supports healing from trauma

KIDNEY 15

- Regulates intestines and lower jiao (diarrhea/constipation, dysmenorrhea, lumbar pain)
- Nourishes Kidneys and yin—most commonly used in Yin Qiao Mai
- Supports healing from trauma

KIDNEY 16

- Regulates qi, alleviates pain
- Regulates and warms intestines (diarrhea/constipation, borborygmus, vomiting, leaky gut syndrome, lin syndrome)
- Treats epigastric distention, pain or cold, shan disorder
- Nourishes Kidneys and yin—most commonly used in Yin Qiao Mai
- Supports healing from trauma
- Strengthens vitality of entire system

KIDNEY 17

- Dispels accumulation and alleviates pain
- Harmonizes the Stomach (abdominal masses, intestinal pain with lack of appetite, diarrhea/constipation, vomiting)
- Regulates and supports the Spleen (great for Earth CF—five element)
- Can be used in combination with **KI11** to strongly support Stomach/Spleen dynamic
- Treats blood in cases of depression/resignation—boosts mood; use this point to manage difficult emotions that may arise in the context of eight extraordinary vessel treatments
- Treats kidney stones and gallstones

KIDNEY 18

- Regulates lower jiao, alleviates pain (dark urine)
- Regulates qi, moves blood stasis (malign blood in uterus, infertility)
- Treats damp conditions in the middle jiao; assists the Spleen to move dampness
- Harmonizes the Stomach/Spleen with the Liver and subdues rebellious qi (digestive issues)

- Overcomes inability to concentrate, foggy mind

- Helps break down the barriers/obstacles an individual has created due to habitual tendencies (self-sabotage)

- Unlocks gates to allow person to step into their power and get out of their own way

- Soothes fear of one's own power/potential

- Treats kidney stones and gallstones

KIDNEY 19

- Regulates qi; subdues rebellious qi to stop cough and wheezing

- Treats fullness and agitation below the Heart

- Disperses malign blood in uterus, treats infertility

- Treats damp conditions in the middle jiao

- Harmonizes the Stomach/Spleen with the Liver and addresses rebellious qi (digestive issues)

- Overcomes inability to concentrate, foggy mind

- Helps break down the barriers/obstacles an individual has created due to habitual tendencies (self-sabotage)

- Unlocks gates to allow person to step into their power and get out of their own way

- Soothes fear of one's own power/potential

- Can be used in combination with **KI20** to help person ease transition

- Treats blood-related Spleen issues

KIDNEY 20

- Harmonizes the Stomach/Spleen with the Liver and subdues rebellious qi (digestive issues)

- Unbinds the chest and transforms phlegm

- Overcomes inability to concentrate, foggy mind

- Prevents palpitations, epilepsy, sudden loss of voice, deviation of the mouth, inability to turn the neck, protrusion or swelling of the tongue

- Helps break down the barriers/obstacles an individual has created due to habitual tendencies (self-sabotage)

- Unlocks gates to allow person to step into their power and get out of their own way

- Soothes fear of one's own power/potential

- Removes gui

- Can be used in combination with **KI19** to help person ease transition

KIDNEY 21

- Fortifies the Spleen (loss of appetite)

- Harmonizes the Stomach/Spleen with the Liver and addresses rebellious qi (digestive issues); stops vomiting

- Benefits the chest and breasts (cough, coughing blood, breast abscess, breast milk not flowing), alleviates pain

- Overcomes inability to concentrate, foggy mind, poor memory

- Helps break down the barriers/obstacles an individual has created due to habitual tendencies (self-sabotage)

- Unlocks gates to allow person to step into their power and get out of their own way

- Soothes fear of one's own power/potential

- Removes gui

- Can be used in cases when patient may need a buffer to emotional turmoil that arises during treatment; treats emotional turmoil

STOMACH 30

- Regulates qi in the lower jiao

- Regulates the Chong Mai

- Subdues running piglet qi and rebellious qi

- Supports post-natal qi

- Treats issues due to undernourishment and supports digestive system

SPLEEN 12

- Invigorates blood, regulates qi, and alleviates pain

- Subdues rebellious qi of the Chong Mai

- Drains damp, clears heat, and regulates urination

The second Chong Mai trajectory (Figure 5.7) travels through the upper part of the vessel and influences speech, throat, and mouth issues; it can often be beneficial for those who have a difficult time in speaking from the heart. Patients may report pressure in the chest or difficulty breathing, and when they go to speak, find it hard to formulate words. This generally reflects deep emotional issues. This particular trajectory is beneficial in addressing eating disorders, especially in adolescents and young adults, as well as asthma. Lastly, this pathway possesses a stronger connection between jing and the spirit of the person and can therefore be beneficial for treating various types of shen disturbances.

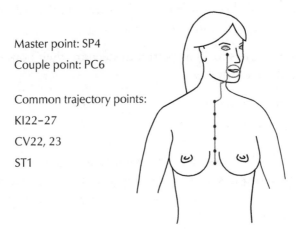

Master point: SP4
Couple point: PC6

Common trajectory points:
KI22–27
CV22, 23
ST1

Figure 5.7 Chong Mai—Second Trajectory

Trajectory Points (Second Trajectory)

Kidney 22–27

Conception Vessel 22 and 23

Stomach 1

KIDNEY 22

- Unbinds the chest

- Subdues rebellious Lung and Stomach qi

- Provides a sense of stability and security while simultaneously broadening one's horizons

- Opens a person's eyes to what may be possible while supporting and anchoring them in the familiar

KIDNEY 23

- Unbinds the chest; stops cough

- Harmonizes the Stomach and subdues rebellious Lung and Stomach qi

- Benefits the breasts

- Provides clarity regarding one's uniqueness and value

- Supports the integration of one's sense of self

KIDNEY 24

- Unbinds the chest, descends Lung qi

- Subdues rebellious Lung and Stomach qi

- Benefits the breasts

- Smooths the flow of Liver qi

- Reignites the spirit in cases of depression

- Soothes deep fears and nightmares

- Clears out the cobwebs of resignation to make room for the wisdom and flow of life

KIDNEY 25

- Unbinds the chest, descends Lung qi

- Subdues rebellious Lung and Stomach qi

- Treats worry, anxiety, and insomnia, especially when the patient is very depleted

- Strengthens the will

KIDNEY 26

- Unbinds the chest and benefits the breasts

- Transforms phlegm and subdues rebellious Lung and Stomach qi

- Treats asthma; moves obstruction out of chest and throat (patient may constantly be attempting to clear their throat)

- Reminds the patient to appreciate and respect the beauty within self and others

- Supports someone who feels discouraged or is "going through the motions"

KIDNEY 27

- Unbinds the chest, descends Lung qi, and stops cough

- Transforms phlegm and alleviates cough and wheezing

- Harmonizes the Stomach and subdues rebellious qi; stops vomiting

- Treats asthma; moves obstruction out of chest and throat (patient may constantly be attempting to clear their throat)

- Treats burnout, exhaustion, and severe irritability

- Rejuvenates spirit and replenishes energy reserves

CONCEPTION VESSEL 22

- Descends rebellious Lung qi and alleviates cough and wheezing
- Benefits the throat and voice
- Addresses plum pit qi and resolves phlegm
- Supports the breath and clarifies the voice
- Treats heartbreak; helps person let go; calms the shen
- Restores all yin channels
- Needles in this point are not to be retained; rather, quickly tonified

CONCEPTION VESSEL 23

- Benefits the tongue and speech
- Descends rebellious qi and alleviates cough
- Addresses plum pit qi and other obstructions such as phlegm
- Supports the breath and clarifies the voice
- Treats heartbreak; helps person let go; calms the shen
- Restores all yin channels
- Needles in this point are not to be retained; rather, quickly tonified

STOMACH 1

- Brightens the eyes and stops lacrimation
- Expels wind and clears heat
- Assists with judgment
- Assists in the movement of vision (physiologically, metaphorically)
- Supports the ability to see clearly what lies ahead and digest what is seen
- Opens structure so a person is able to receive, discern, and disseminate the information appropriately

- Is great for someone who has a difficult time with discernment, which can create boundary issues

The third trajectory (Figure 5.8) within the Chong Mai is most beneficial for treating conditions related to damp-heat in the lower jiao, such as bowel syndromes, genital concerns (sexually transmitted diseases), and menstrual cycle syndromes. This particular pathway helps more with physical symptoms, as opposed to emotional distress. However, it is best to not separate the physical from the emotional and/or spiritual bodies of an individual. There will be spiritual movement in the person regardless of which vessel is treated. This trajectory has a direct relationship to the Liver meridian and can be used in treating conditions associated with Hun disturbances, especially if the patient is experiencing nightmares.

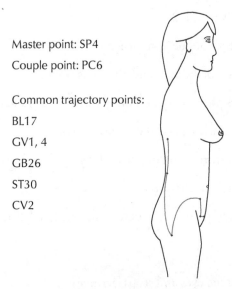

Master point: SP4

Couple point: PC6

Common trajectory points:

BL17

GV1, 4

GB26

ST30

CV2

Figure 5.8 Chong Mai—Third Trajectory

Trajectory Points (Third Trajectory)

Stomach 30

Gallbladder 26

Conception Vessel 2

Governor Vessel 1 (but can substitute GV4)

Bladder 17

STOMACH 30

- Regulates qi in the lower jiao
- Regulates the Chong Mai
- Subdues running piglet qi and rebellious qi
- Supports post-natal qi
- Treats issues due to undernourishment and supports digestive system

GALLBLADDER 26

- Resolves dampness in the lower jiao
- Regulates the Dai Mai and the uterus; regulates menstruation and stops leukorrhea
- Activates the channel and alleviates pain

CONCEPTION VESSEL 2

- Benefits the Bladder and regulates urination
- Regulates lower jiao
- Warms and invigorates the Kidneys; consolidates the essence

GOVERNOR VESSEL 1 (CAN SUBSTITUTE GV4)

- Regulates Du Mai and Ren Mai
- Resolves dampness
- Benefits the two lower orifices (treats hemorrhoids)
- Activates the channel and alleviates pain
- Calms the spirit and opens the mind's orifices
- Extinguishes interior wind

BLADDER 17

- Invigorates blood and dispels stasis

- Cools blood heat and stops bleeding

- Nourishes and harmonizes the blood and qi

- Unbinds the chest, harmonizes the diaphragm, and descends rebellious qi

- Benefits the sinews

- Can be combined with **CV2** and **GV4** for prolapse

Possible Off-Trajectory Points
LOWER SPLEEN COMMAND POINTS

Using points on the Spleen meridian while treating the Chong Mai offers a unique quality to the treatments overall. While initially it is best to open the Chong Mai by itself, after treating the Chong Mai three times using trajectory points, one can embark upon a more advanced treatment of the Chong Mai using Spleen command points. This is a wonderful option for treating the Chong Mai on the third trajectory for the purpose of supporting the lower limbs (e.g., restless legs, weak limbs, varicose veins in the legs, general fatigue, "weak in the knees").

It may be difficult to decide which of the command points to use, so there is a general guide to follow when determining the best selection of points.

While treating the Chong Mai, and after treating it traditionally, at least three times as outlined in this book, make your selection of Spleen points as follows:

- If interested in treating based on the season: **SP1** for Spring, **SP2** for Summer, **SP3** for Late Summer, **SP5** for Fall and **SP9** for Winter.

- If interested in assisting with clarity, ambition, direction, and vision (both physically as well as metaphorically), combine **SP1** with **SP6**.

- For fertility, add **SP8** and **SP9**. To help sustain pregnancy, add **SP4**.

- For deep depression, combine **SP5** with **SP6**. If Yin is deficient, add **SP9**.

- If there are significant digestive issues, combine **SP7** with **SP6**, and add **SP2** if the digestive issues also include epigastric issues.

- These Spleen points are beneficial for lethargy, fatigue, appetite issues, and digestive problems. They nourish the blood and support the blood vessels with circulation and containment.

The fourth and fifth trajectories (Figure 5.9) within the Chong Mai have a close relationship with the Qiao Mai, starting in the pelvic region and traveling down into the foot. Treating these pathways can be beneficial for patients who stand for long periods of time (e.g., cashiers, hairdressers, waiters). Over time, these individuals can develop pain in the lower back or abdomen, as well as physiological conditions associated with the feet such as plantar fasciitis, stress fractures in the feet, or any kind of foot pain in general. It is beneficial to treat these pathways for chronic pain in the areas of the pelvic cavity and down the medial aspect of the lower limbs and feet. Both trajectories have a strong relationship with the Spleen and Stomach, and are therefore useful with digestive issues. Lastly, these trajectories are considered supporting pathways to the Chong Mai in general, meaning they can be coupled with other Chong Mai trajectories. This will be explained further in Chapter 12.

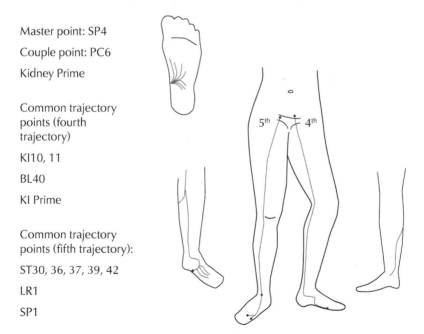

Master point: SP4

Couple point: PC6

Kidney Prime

Common trajectory points (fourth trajectory)

KI10, 11

BL40

KI Prime

Common trajectory points (fifth trajectory):

ST30, 36, 37, 39, 42

LR1

SP1

5th   4th

Figure 5.9 Chong Mai—Fourth and Fifth Trajectories

Trajectory Points (Fourth Trajectory)

Kidney Prime (bottom of the foot at the arch; lateral and distal 1 cun to Kidney 2)

Kidney 3–6, 10, and 11

Bladder 40

KIDNEY PRIME

- Prepare the patient and use a small-gauge needle because this is often painful

- Can be used with moxa direct on the foot or moxa on the needle

Kidney Prime is located on the bottom of the foot, 2.5 cun medial to Kidney 2, and 3 cun distal to the calcaneus. It is referred to as Kidney Prime because it precedes Kidney 1.

From a physical standpoint, it is helpful with plantar fasciitis, plantar warts, heel pain, and any issues related to the bottom of the foot. It can be added to other treatment strategies for issues concerning the Achilles tendon.

It lends tremendous support for grounding and encourages the meridian system to use resources efficiently and effectively. From a mental and emotional perspective, it can be effective for treating depression (especially when combined with Kidney 1). Kidney Prime treats leg pain that is medial in its pain trajectory and provides support to the immune system, fertility and reproductive organs, and the Kidneys. It has a direct line to the pelvic cavity and lower jiao.

KIDNEY 3

- Nourishes Kidney yin and clears deficiency heat

- Tonifies Kidney yang

- Grasps the qi and benefits the Lung

- Calms the spirit

- Benefits the essence

- Strengthens the lumbar spine and knees

- Regulates the uterus

KIDNEY 4

- Reinforces the Kidneys
- Grasps the qi and benefits the Lung
- Calms the spirit, strengthens the will, and dispels fear
- Benefits urination
- Strengthens the back

KIDNEY 5

- Benefits urination
- Regulates the Chong Mai and Ren Mai
- Regulates the uterus and menstruation

KIDNEY 6

- Nourishes Kidney yin and clears deficiency heat
- Benefits the eyes
- Invigorates the Yin Qiao Mai
- Calms the spirit
- Benefits the throat
- Regulates the lower jiao, uterus, and menstruation

KIDNEY 10

- Resolves dampness and clears damp-heat from the lower jiao
- Nourishes Kidney yin
- Activates the channel and alleviates pain
- Can treat with moxa on the needle

KIDNEY 11

- Benefits and regulates the lower jiao (seminal emissions, impotence, exhaustion of five zang, enuresis, lin syndrome, painful genitals, vaginismus, shan disorder)

- Resolves dampness and clears heat

- Treats extreme/acute pelvic disorders such as prolapse or cancers in the pelvic cavity in both females and males (prostate, uterine, etc.)

- Can be used in combination: Yin Qiao Mai + Chong Mai + **KI11** for fertility; also supports the Stomach and resolves damp conditions

- Can be used with **KI13** for herpes

BLADDER 40

- Benefits the lumbar region and knees

- Activates the channel and alleviates pain

- Clears heat and cools the blood

- Clears summer-heat and stops vomiting and diarrhea

- Benefits the Bladder

Off Trajectory Point (Fourth Trajectory)

KIDNEY 9

- Clears the Heart and transforms phlegm; opens the chest

- Calms the spirit and opens the mind's orifices

- Tonifies Kidney yin

- Regulates the Yin Wei Mai

- Regulates qi and alleviates pain

- Helps the person break free from the cycle of obsessiveness about the past (trauma, grief); helps to alleviate anxiety, with moxa on the needle

Trajectory Points (Fifth Trajectory)

Stomach 30, 36, 37, 39, and 42

Spleen 1

Liver 1

STOMACH 30

- Regulates qi in the lower jiao
- Regulates the Chong Mai
- Subdues running piglet qi and rebellious qi
- Supports post-natal qi
- Treats issues due to undernourishment and supports digestive system

STOMACH 36

- Harmonizes the Stomach
- Tonifies the Spleen and resolves dampness; resolves edema
- Supports the upright qi and fosters the original qi
- Tonifies qi and nourishes blood and yin
- Regulates ying–wei qi dynamic
- Clears fire and calms the spirit
- Activates the channel and alleviates pain
- Raises the yang and restores consciousness
- Treats issues due to undernourishment and supports digestive system

- Regulates the intestines
- Brightens the eyes

STOMACH 37

- Regulates the Stomach and intestines; resolves food stagnation
- Clears damp-heat and alleviates diarrhea and dysentery
- Regulates the Spleen and Stomach
- Subdues rebellious qi
- Activates the channel and alleviates pain
- Treats blood stagnation

STOMACH 39

- Regulates Small Intestine qi and transforms stagnation
- Regulates and harmonizes the intestines and clears damp-heat
- Eliminates wind-damp
- Activates the channel and alleviates pain
- Treats blood stagnation

STOMACH 42

- Regulates the intestines
- Clears heat from the Stomach channel
- Harmonizes the Stomach fu
- Tonifies the Stomach and Spleen
- Calms the spirit; opens the mind's orifices
- Activates the channel and alleviates pain
- Treats issues due to undernourishment and supports digestive system

SPLEEN 1

- Stops bleeding
- Regulates the Spleen
- Unbinds the chest
- Calms the Heart and spirit, and restores consciousness

LIVER 1

- Regulates Liver qi and menstruation
- Resolves damp-heat in the genitals and Bladder
- Regulates qi in the lower jiao, treats shan disorder and alleviates pain
- Revives consciousness and calms the spirit

Disharmonies of the Chong Mai

When the Chong Mai is not fully open and functioning, the patient suffers from disharmony within the vessel. This can be expressed physically, emotionally, or spiritually. Because the body is multi-dimensional, when one level of existence is impacted, all three levels are affected. While disharmonies among the eight extraordinary vessels may share symptoms and syndromes, some are more specific to the Chong Mai, such as intergenerational imprinting, fatalistic thinking, an inability to truly see reality, and living with some degree of delusion and distress. Other more shared symptoms include depression, fear, anger, worry, obsessive compulsive disorder, and addictions.

A person with Chong Mai disharmony finds it difficult to take in new ideas, often has long-standing abuse issues, is easily exhausted, and is significantly impacted by their afflictive emotions. They can express nervous energy when discussing emotional topics, may worry excessively about mundane activities, and usually have a more introverted personality. It is difficult for them to take a leap of faith with new endeavors or relationships, express appropriate emotions, and articulate what they are feeling.

The Chong Mai is useful in treating gynecological disorders, digestive issues, prolapse, and pathology of the Heart. An imbalance in the Chong Mai significantly impacts a person's ability to possess self-acceptance and self-love. For this reason, the Chong Mai is helpful in supporting transgender patients, via the aligning effects of finding comfort and ease in one's physical body.

Alignment of the Chong Mai could be equated to alignment in the Kidney–Heart axis. In the classical texts, there is reference to an appropriate presence of heat in the lower jiao which is referred to as "wisdom fire." As the pathway of the Chong Mai ascends in the body, moving upwards through the three jiaos, the heat becomes lighter. The Central Channel in the body is associated with the Kidney, Spleen, and Liver meridians.

In addition to the previously mentioned psycho-spiritual symptoms, treatment on the Chong Mai can address fertility, pelvic cavity syndromes, low libido, and Kidney-related pathology in the deep pathways. Treating the Chong Mai will release muscle memory trapped in the body, ease mental restlessness, and treat digestive issues, specifically rebellious qi. It affects the Heart, chest, and Stomach (the Stomach assists in our ability to take in new ideas), and plays a critical role in an individual achieving their destiny. It regulates the flow of qi and blood in the twelve primary meridians.

It is important to remember the spirit of the points on the various Chong Mai pathways. A good understanding of the spirit of the points will help in determining which pathway to set with intention, as well as the point selection. It is important to remember even if the intention is to treat the physiological condition of the individual, the emotional and spirit body will be impacted; therefore, it is wise to consider the spirit and disposition of the individual to ensure they have the stability needed to benefit from these deep vessels.

The Chong Mai is the Central Channel of an individual. Keep in mind that the Central Channel possesses essence qi from the Kidneys, the individual's ability to achieve in a particular lifetime, and not only speak from the Heart, but live up to the potential destined for an individual with utmost authenticity. In working with any of the eight extraordinary vessels, the practitioner will awaken the spirit, and this is especially true of the Chong Mai, so it is important to be mindful as a practitioner. The patient may feel as if they have awakened from a deep slumber; therefore, this should be done with care.

REN MAI

Master point: LU7

Couple point: KI6

Common trajectory points:
CV1–24

Second trajectory through
the face ending at ST1

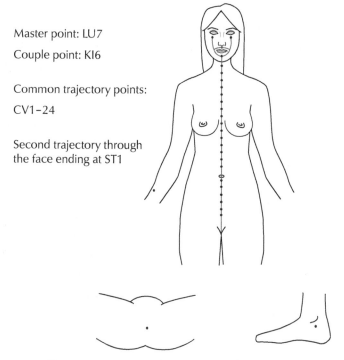

Figure 5.10 Ren Mai (Directing Vessel, Sea of Yin)

Master Point: Lung 7

Couple Point: Kidney 6

An individual's ability to bond with other beings is a reflection of the health and vitality of the Ren Mai. The number-one indicator of Ren Mai health is understanding how the patient bonds with children, partners, friends, family, and strangers. This vessel is most active at birth when the baby is given (or not) to its mother, and how the baby experiences those first few moments of life, breathing on its own and being held. The development of the Ren Mai is lifelong; however, its most active period is from birth to about the age of nine for most people. Once an individual reaches the age of nine, their *style* of bonding with other beings becomes more established.

Babies not born into loving and nourishing families suffer greatly from the inability to have healthy relationships in their adult lives. If the disharmony goes untreated, an individual will suffer an entire life of difficult relationships because they never developed the ability to bond with other beings in a healthy way. The Ren Mai allows us to bear the burden of being human, to take charge of our lives, to be responsible, and to cope at each level of existence (body, mind, spirit). The Ren Mai allows us to have profound reverence for our own lives, as well as the lives of others.

Over the course of one's life, multiple traumas can greatly impact the health of the individual's Ren Mai. With each perceived traumatic experience, the Ren Mai takes a hit and, in cases where there is pre-existing disharmony, is unable to appropriately readjust to life. This can lead to panic attacks, phobias, mood disorders, and feeling ungrounded. In extreme cases, there is a complete disconnection from spirituality, or a lack of nurturance coupled with extreme grief and fear.

People who are involved with the legal system for consistently breaking laws likely harbour deep pathology in the Ren Mai. This is because they have a difficult time honoring their life as well as the lives of others. The deeper the imbalance in the Ren Mai, the more extreme the criminal behavior.

Treating the Ren Mai can help ground the spirit of the Liver and the Hun, and return balance. It does this by working with the Chong Mai to restore spiritual equilibrium. The Chong Mai and the Ren Mai work closely together to help achieve the potential spiritual awareness of the person. There are many things that can cause "spiritual deficiency." If the pathology is one of a spiritual nature rather than physical or emotional, pairing the Chong Mai and the Ren Mai will help propel the patient forward in terms of spiritual development and awareness.

Although the opening points for the Ren Mai are located on the Lung and Kidney channels, the trajectory points are located on the Conception Vessel (CV) meridian. The trajectory travels up the midline of the torso, and the deeper trajectory encircles the mouth and goes into the eyes, known as the "Great Thoroughfare," later referred to as Ren Mai.

The Ren Mai receives and transports qi of all the yin meridians (Heart, Pericardium, Spleen, Lung, Kidney, and Liver). Therefore, it regulates organs and organ systems associated with these officials (e.g., menstruation, asthma, respiratory syndromes, matters of the Heart, and body fluids). Remember to evaluate the disharmony observed in the patient from a broad perspective. Treating the Ren Mai is essentially treating all five yin officials and their respective meridians. In most cases, individuals have mixed and multiple conditions; therefore, it is important to evaluate the person on all three levels of existence. For example, symptomatology may take the form of anxiousness, irritability, fragility, addictions, difficulty bonding, stunted spirituality, and chronic panic attacks. These symptoms would be cause to consider treating the Ren Mai, along with pulse and tongue diagnosis to support the decision.

Additionally, treating the Ren Mai can ground the ethereal soul of the patient because the Chong Mai and the Ren Mai work closely together to substantiate a person's potential for spiritual awareness. If the patient's greatest pathology is rooted in spiritual deficiency, this may be a treatment to consider in advanced treatment planning. There may be situations when the Ren Mai is in acute distress, which is often grief related. A sudden shock, specifically the unexpected death of a loved one, can cause an acute disturbance of the Ren Mai. Fear can also be an issue that impacts the Ren Mai; such is the case with veterans who have been exposed to the horrors of combat.

Naturally, treating the Ren Mai with acupuncture can be beneficial, but other kinds of therapy, such as yoga, breathing exercises, and, of course, talk therapy, in addition to acupuncture can offer a synergistic effect. Opening the channels in the body specific to the Lung can offer relief to the patient in letting go enough to expand the breath. Doing this repeatedly can give the person grounding to cope with the sudden traumatic event.

When setting intention for accessing the Ren Mai, think of all that is yin. The best way to positively impact the Ren Mai is through activating the channel with the MP and CP, and trajectory points on the CV meridian. Other theories suggest GV points; however, there may be more clarity of intention when simply treating the Ren Mai with respective trajectory points on the CV line.

Treating the Ren Mai supports the shen and anchors yang. In extreme cases of Ren Mai disturbance, the yang can become ungrounded, possibly collapsed. Treating the Ren Mai supports both the yin and the yang by realigning and supporting yin, and anchoring yang and shen. This also explains how treating the Ren Mai can be supportive for those with addictions or recovering from cancer treatments.

Disharmonies of the Ren Mai

If the treatment strategy is to address a spiritual deficiency, accessing upper CV points starting at CV14 can bring tremendous benefit, especially if they are conjunct Heart/Pericardium issues. Treating upper Kidney points can also be a beneficial strategy. However, if the deficiency is deeper and more work is needed, opening the Ren Mai, and adding CV trajectory points can allow the patient to delve deeper into their life's work (purpose). Using CV14 and 15 initially can help stabilize the Heart and shen. Consider employing upper CV or Kidney points when addressing symptoms of an emotional nature such as grief, fear, anxiousness, and sadness.

There are a couple more classic symptoms related specifically to disharmony of the Ren Mai, including a strong tendency toward addictions, inappropriate laughter, and phobias. Panic attacks can be treated by both the Chong Mai and Ren Mai. Phobias, however, are more specific to Ren Mai.

In viewing an individual from a yin/yang perspective, if yin deficiency is present, yang most likely needs anchoring. Treating yin creates a healing shift and helps to anchor yang and settle the shen. Treating the Ren Mai will help warm the interior, expel cold and damp, promote descending of Lung qi, support the Kidneys receiving qi, and transform body fluids.

Should there be long-standing disharmony within the Ren Mai, yin becomes more deficient, yang begins to collapse, yin and yang start to separate, and the person becomes more ungrounded. This is reflected in multiple symptoms on all three levels of existence: physical, emotional, and spiritual.

Although treating the Ren Mai does address the body fluids and blood, it primarily addresses qi. The Ren Mai, like all the extraordinary vessels, has a close relationship to the Triple Energizer meridian, helping to facilitate communication among all the officials in the body.

Trajectory Points

Conception Vessel 1–24

Stomach 1 and 4

QUICK REFERENCE OVERVIEW

- **Conception Vessels 1–15** address deficiency at large
- **Conception Vessels 16–22** address stasis at large
- **Conception Vessels 23 and 24** are the meeting point of the midline and connecting point of Yin linking vessels

CONCEPTION VESSEL 1

- Regulates the two lower orifices and resolves dampness
- Drains damp-heat
- Calms the spirit
- Promotes resuscitation and revives from drowning

CONCEPTION VESSEL 2

- Benefits the Bladder and regulates urination
- Regulates lower jiao
- Warms and invigorates the Kidneys; consolidates the essence

CONCEPTION VESSEL 3

- Benefits the Bladder, regulates qi transformation, and drains damp-heat
- Resolves dampness and treats leukorrhea
- Benefits the uterus and regulates menstruation
- Dispels stagnation and benefits the lower jiao
- Nourishes the Kidneys and essence

CONCEPTION VESSEL 4

- Benefits the original qi and essence
- Nourishes blood and yin

- Tonifies and nourishes the Kidneys; supports Kidneys in grasping the qi

- Warms and fortifies the Spleen

- Benefits the uterus, assists conception, and regulates menstruation

- Subdues rebellious qi in the Chong Mai

- Regulates the lower jiao and benefits the Bladder

- Regulates Small Intestine qi

- Restores collapse

- Roots the shen and the Hun

CONCEPTION VESSEL 5

- Opens and benefits the water passages for transformation of fluids in the lower jiao

- Regulates qi and alleviates pain in the lower jiao

- Regulates the uterus

- Tonifies original qi

CONCEPTION VESSEL 6

- Tonifies original qi

- Tonifies qi and yang

- Tonifies the Kidneys

- Rescues collapse of yang; raises sinking qi

- Regulates qi and harmonizes blood, especially in the lower jiao

- Treats yin stasis; treats slack yin

CONCEPTION VESSEL 7

- Regulates the uterus and menstruation

- Regulates the Chong Mai

- Resolves dampness in the lower jiao

- Nourishes yin

- Benefits the lower abdomen and genital region

- Can be paired with **CV9** for fertility

- Supports yin, increases fluid secretions; tills and fertilizes the soil of fertility

CONCEPTION VESSEL 8 (NOT NEEDLED)

- Warms the yang and rescues collapse

- Tonifies the Spleen and original qi

- Warms and harmonizes the intestines

- Is centering

CONCEPTION VESSEL 9

- Opens and regulates the water passages and treats edema

- Harmonizes the intestines and dispels accumulation

- Can be paired with **CV7** for fertility

- Supports yin, increases fluid secretions; tills and fertilizes the soil of fertility

CONCEPTION VESSEL 10

- Harmonizes the Stomach and regulates qi

- Resolves food stagnation

- Treats eating disorders, addresses metabolism problems

CONCEPTION VESSEL 11

- Harmonizes the middle jiao and regulates qi

- Supports the functions of the Stomach

CONCEPTION VESSEL 12

- Harmonizes the middle jiao and subdues rebellious qi
- Tonifies the Stomach and Spleen
- Resolves dampness and phlegm
- Regulates qi and alleviates pain
- Treats digestive issues
- Helps with movement of fluids and blood
- Calms the spirit; centering

CONCEPTION VESSEL 13

- Harmonizes the Stomach and regulates qi
- Descends rebellious Stomach qi and alleviates vomiting
- Regulates the Heart

CONCEPTION VESSEL 14

- Regulates Heart qi and alleviates pain
- Descends Lung qi and unbinds the chest
- Calms the spirit and opens the mind's orifices; transforms phlegm
- Harmonizes the Stomach and subdues rebellious qi

CONCEPTION VESSEL 15

- Calms the spirit and opens the mind's orifices
- Descends Lung qi and unbinds the chest; regulates the Heart
- Supports interpersonal relationships; relaxes and opens the chest
- Accesses ancestral qi
- Treats upper respiratory issues
- Treats pectus excavatum (condition with concave sternum and flared ribcage causing shortness of breath and chest pain)

CONCEPTION VESSEL 16

- Unbinds the chest

- Regulates the Stomach and descends rebellious qi

- Supports interpersonal relationships; relaxes and opens the chest

- Accesses ancestral qi

- Treats upper respiratory issues

- Treats pectus excavatum (condition with concave sternum and flared ribcage causing shortness of breath and chest pain)

CONCEPTION VESSEL 17

- Unbinds the chest and regulates qi

- Descends rebellion of Lung and Stomach

- Tonifies the gathering qi

- Benefits the breasts and promotes lactation

- Supports interpersonal relationships; relaxes and opens the chest

- Accesses ancestral qi

- Treats upper respiratory issues

- Treats pectus excavatum (condition with concave sternum and flared ribcage causing shortness of breath and chest pain)

CONCEPTION VESSEL 18

- Unbinds the chest

- Regulates and descends qi

CONCEPTION VESSEL 19

- Unbinds the chest

- Regulates and descends qi

CONCEPTION VESSEL 20

- Unbinds the chest

- Regulates and descends qi

- Addresses plum pit qi and other obstructions such as phlegm

CONCEPTION VESSEL 21

- Descends Stomach qi and dispels food accumulation

- Unbinds the chest and descends Lung qi

- Benefits the throat

- Addresses plum pit qi and other obstructions such as phlegm

CONCEPTION VESSEL 22

- Descends rebellious Lung qi and alleviates cough and wheezing

- Benefits the throat and voice

- Addresses plum pit qi and resolves phlegm

- Supports the breath and clarifies the voice

- Treats heartbreak; helps person let go; calms the shen

- Restores all yin channels

- Needles in this point are not to be retained; rather, quickly tonified

CONCEPTION VESSEL 23

- Benefits the tongue and speech

- Descends rebellious qi and alleviates cough

- Addresses plum pit qi and other obstructions such as phlegm

- Supports the breath and clarifies the voice

- Treats heartbreak; helps person let go; calms the shen

- Restores all yin channels

- Needles in this point are not to be retained; rather, quickly tonified

CONCEPTION VESSEL 24

- Extinguishes wind and benefits the face
- Regulates the Conception Vessel

STOMACH 1

- Brightens the eyes and stops lacrimation
- Expels wind and clears heat
- Assists with judgment
- Assists in the movement of vision (physiologically, metaphorically)
- Supports the ability to see clearly what lies ahead and digest what is seen
- Opens structure so a person is able to receive, discern, and disseminate the information appropriately
- Is great for someone who has a difficult time with discernment, which can create boundary issues

STOMACH 4

- Expels wind from the face; treats acne
- Activates the channel and alleviates pain
- Treats eating disorders, addresses metabolism problems
- Assists with judgment
- Assists in the movement of vision (physiologically, metaphorically)
- Supports the ability to see clearly what lies ahead and digest what is seen
- Opens structure so a person is able to receive, discern, and disseminate the information appropriately

- Is great for someone who has a difficult time with discernment, which can create boundary issues

To discern between pathology in the Chong Mai or the Ren Mai, look at the whole landscape and observe the larger picture. Remember, there is essentially no right or wrong in choosing between these two vessels. Ultimately, in most cases the patient will need both vessels treated. In Chapter 4 there is a clear, more detailed method of discerning which vessel to start with when treating patients.

Remember the body is wise, and simply activating the vessel with the MP and CP alone is a powerful and beneficial treatment. Never underestimate the profundity of simply activating the vessel.

DU MAI

Master point: SI3

Couple point: BL62

Common trajectory points:
GV1–28

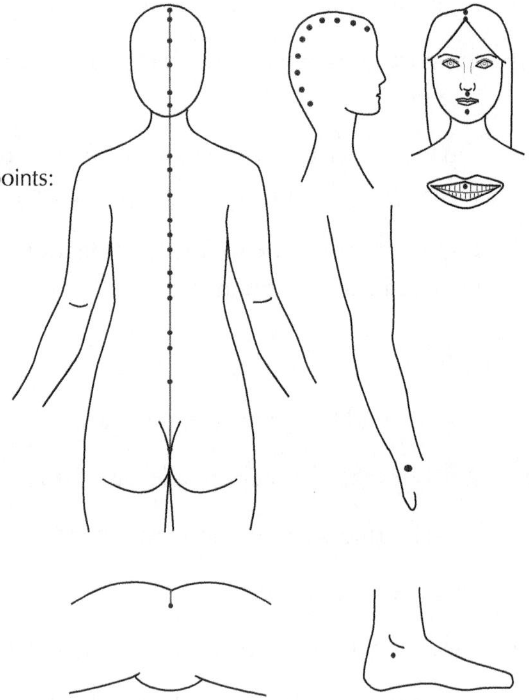

Figure 5.11 Du Mai (Sea of Yang)

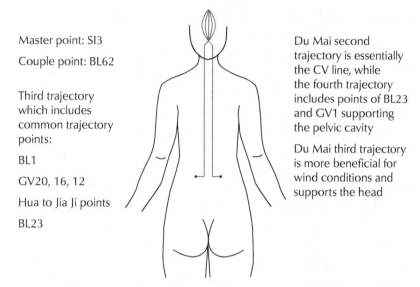

Master point: SI3

Couple point: BL62

Third trajectory
which includes
common trajectory
points:

BL1

GV20, 16, 12

Hua to Jia Ji points

BL23

Du Mai second
trajectory is essentially
the CV line, while
the fourth trajectory
includes points of BL23
and GV1 supporting
the pelvic cavity

Du Mai third trajectory
is more beneficial for
wind conditions and
supports the head

Figure 5.12 Du Mai—Second and Third Trajectories

Master Point: Small Intestine 3

Couple Point: Bladder 62

All the polarities that exist in life fall under the domain of the Du Mai. Du Mai and Ren Mai are synonymous with fire and water, above and below. It is the spine and the corresponding deep vessel that allow for the breath to ascend and descend correctly in the wake of spiritual growth. Breath and breathing techniques, especially associated with meditation, are linked to the health of the Du Mai. In meditation, the back must be tall and straight, unlocking the blockages of the Du Mai. The deep breath which stretches the Du Mai is what is referred to as "true breath." It is the deeper breath within the body, initiating at the meeting point of Ren Mai and Du Mai deep inside the pelvic cavity. Ren Mai and Du Mai work closely together, though they are separate deep vessels, yin and yang respectively.

Experienced meditators can activate the Du Mai through breathing techniques. There is a Microcosmic Orbit that arises from the place where the body meets the earth in meditation, at the perineum. The Du Mai is a highly spiritual vessel and allows the space needed for humans to connect with their higher selves, and ultimately achieve spiritual awakening.

Directing the activities of the body, mind, and spirit, the Du Mai functions as the Governor to the Emperor (the Heart), watching over the kingdom with love and wisdom that is directed from the Heart. In fact, the Heart, brain, and Kidneys are profoundly impacted by the Du Mai. Although the mind is housed in the Heart, its foundation is in the Kidney essence. Therefore, the relationship between the Heart and Kidneys can also be accessed via the Du Mai. This is especially true in the treatment of emotions and emotional pathology, most notably depression.

On a physical level, activating the Du Mai is useful in treating issues within the pelvic cavity. Its primary trajectory begins just behind the umbilicus. Given that it travels through the pelvic cavity and up the back, it is beneficial for treating renal symptoms, infertility, incontinence, chronic back aches, and heaviness in the head, headaches, and various kinds of Heart pain. The Du Mai is used to raise yang and support and strengthen the patient's backbone physically and metaphorically. Slack yang and tense yin pathology manifest as prolapse.

Treatment on the Du Mai helps a person practice control over their mind, rather than feeling at the mercy of their thoughts. When there is pathology in the Du Mai, regardless of how subtle or gross, the individual feels overwhelmed and hopeless regarding their ability to survive. Treating this vessel can help settle the Corporeal Soul, the Po. Although the Po is often thought of as more yin, in terms of its essences it is more yang. Therefore, treating the Du Mai helps settle conditions relating to the Corporeal Soul (Lung—breath, Large Intestine—letting go). The ascending and descending of qi in the Du Mai makes a unique energetic route in the body that has a profound impact on all three levels of existence.

Disharmonies of the Du Mai include anxiousness (Heart), fear (Kidney), agitation, anger (Liver), and qi stagnation (pervasive). These symptoms may manifest as a lack of determination and ambition, difficulty completing tasks or participating in teamwork, mental inflexibility, narrow-mindedness or stubbornness, a "spineless" disposition, or a tendency to be over-controlling. Treating the Du Mai will help settle the Corporeal Soul, support physical issues related to the spine and brain, and help heal trauma housed in the pelvic cavity.

The Du Mai is associated with being upright, and the energy both ascends and descends through the Du Mai. This makes the trajectory beneficial in treating wind conditions as well as neurological conditions.

It can be used to treat gait abnormalities, walking, spinal rigidity, and balance. From a spiritual standpoint, it is associated with the ego and perception of duality (subject and object).

In select cases of serious neurological distress, after activating the Du Mai and selecting trajectory points, consider an alternative approach: since trajectory points are typically needled bilaterally, the chosen Governor Vessel points may be needled to both sides of the spine, directing the needle toward the midline. This must be done with caution, given the degree of innervation on the spine.

The first trajectory is the primary trajectory, which includes all points on the Governor Vessel. While there are three other trajectories according to the theory, the first trajectory can be used to treat any disharmonies associated with the Du Mai.

Trajectory Points

Governor Vessel 1–28

GOVERNOR VESSEL 1 (CAN SUBSTITUTE GV4)

- Regulates Du Mai and Ren Mai
- Resolves dampness
- Benefits the two lower orifices (treats hemorrhoids)
- Activates the channel and alleviates pain
- Calms the spirit and opens the mind's orifices
- Extinguishes interior wind

GOVERNOR VESSEL 2

- Extinguishes interior wind
- Benefits the lumbar region and legs
- Dispels wind-damp

GOVERNOR VESSEL 3

- Tonifies yang
- Dispels wind-damp
- Benefits the lumbar region and legs
- Regulates the lower jiao
- Treats fertility issues and dispels cold in pelvic cavity

GOVERNOR VESSEL 4

- Tonifies Kidney yang and warms Ming Men
- Tonifies the original qi
- Expels cold
- Clears heat
- Tonifies and regulates the Du Mai
- Tonifies the Kidneys and essence
- Benefits the lumbar spine (treats lower back pain)
- Clears the mind
- Extinguishes interior wind

GOVERNOR VESSEL 5

- Benefits the lumbar spine (treats lower back pain)
- Benefits the lower jiao

GOVERNOR VESSEL 6

- Fortifies the Spleen and drains damp
- Benefits the spine

GOVERNOR VESSEL 7

- Benefits the spine
- Benefits the middle jiao

GOVERNOR VESSEL 8

- Extinguishes interior wind and relaxes the sinews
- Soothes the Liver, pacifies wind, and relieves spasm
- Calms the spirit

GOVERNOR VESSEL 9

- Regulates the Liver and Gallbladder
- Fortifies the Spleen, drains dampness, and regulates the middle jiao
- Resolves damp-heat (jaundice)
- Unbinds the chest and opens the diaphragm

GOVERNOR VESSEL 10

- Alleviates cough and wheezing
- Clears heat and detoxifies poison
- Treats mid-back pain
- Calms the spirit, gives breath
- Supports a person's ability to receive new ideas and broadens perspective

GOVERNOR VESSEL 11

- Tonifies the Heart and Lung, and calms the spirit
- Clears heat and extinguishes interior wind
- Treats mid-back pain

GOVERNOR VESSEL 12

- Clears heat from the Lung and Heart
- Calms the spirit and opens the mind's orifices
- Extinguishes interior wind

- Tonifies Lung qi
- Treats upper back pain

GOVERNOR VESSEL 13

- Regulates Shao Yang
- Clears heat and treats malaria
- Regulates the Du Mai
- Treats upper back pain and neck pain

GOVERNOR VESSEL 14

- Expels exterior wind and firms the exterior
- Regulates ying–wei dynamic
- Clears heat and treats malaria
- Tonifies deficiency
- Extinguishes interior wind
- Clears the mind
- Tonifies yang
- Treats neck pain

GOVERNOR VESSEL 15

- Benefits the tongue and treats muteness
- Extinguishes interior wind
- Clears the mind
- Benefits the neck and spine (treats neck pain)
- Assists with the ability to speak one's mind, and speech impediments

GOVERNOR VESSEL 16

- Extinguishes interior wind

- Expels exterior wind

- Nourishes the Sea of Marrow and benefits the brain, head, and neck (treats neck pain)

- Calms the spirit and opens the mind's orifices

GOVERNOR VESSEL 17

- Extinguishes interior wind and alleviates pain (treats neck pain, tremors)

- Benefits the eyes and brain

- Calms the spirit and opens the mind's orifices

GOVERNOR VESSEL 18

- Pacifies wind and alleviates pain (treats tremors)

- Calms the spirit

GOVERNOR VESSEL 19

- Eliminates wind and alleviates pain (treats tremors)

- Calms the spirit and opens the mind's orifices

GOVERNOR VESSEL 20

- Pacifies wind and subdues yang (treats tremors)

- Raises yang and counters prolapse

- Benefits the head and sense organs (opens consciousness, treats numbness and loss of sensation)

- Nourishes the Sea of Marrow

- Benefits the brain and calms the spirit

GOVERNOR VESSEL 21

- Eliminates wind and treats convulsions and tremors
- Benefits the head

ASHI POINT BETWEEN GV21 AND GV22

- Widens the physical span of treatment

GOVERNOR VESSEL 22

- Benefits the nose
- Eliminates wind and benefits the head (treats tremors)

GOVERNOR VESSEL 23

- Benefits the nose and brightens the eyes
- Eliminates wind, benefits the head and face, and dispels swelling
- Calms the spirit

GOVERNOR VESSEL 24

- Calms the spirit and opens the mind's orifices
- Extinguishes internal wind and benefits the head and brain
- Benefits the nose and brightens the eyes

GOVERNOR VESSEL 25

- Benefits the nose

GOVERNOR VESSEL 26

- Restores consciousness; extinguishes interior wind
- Calms the spirit and opens the mind's orifices
- Benefits the face and nose, expels wind
- Benefits the spine and treats acute lumbar sprain

- Regulates the water passages of the upper jiao

- Treats madness and psychiatric disorders

- Quiets a person who tends toward a manic disposition

GOVERNOR VESSEL 27

- Clears heat, generates fluid, and benefits the mouth

- Calms the spirit

- Treats madness and psychiatric disorders

- Quiets a person who tends toward a manic disposition

GOVERNOR VESSEL 28

- Clears heat and benefits the gums

- Benefits the nose and eyes

- Treats madness and psychiatric disorders

- Quiets a person who tends toward a manic disposition

The second trajectory (see Figure 5.12) runs up the anterior midline of the body, and while this is typically seen as the yin side of the body corresponding to the Ren Mai and Conception Vessel meridians, the Du Mai trajectory runs behind the Ren Mai. A profile view would show the second Du Mai trajectory running between the first trajectory of the Du Mai and the Ren Mai, internally deep in the body. The points to access the trajectory are located on the Conception Vessel. This particular trajectory is used to treat issues of spiritual deficiency, which includes a deep depression resulting from the individual's failure to fulfill a spiritual accomplishment. The patient will use similar wording to describe their depression—issues around not fulfilling one's potential spiritually. The Chong Mai, Ren Mai, and Du Mai have meeting points deep in the body at the perineum, and then come together again and intersect in the throat and mouth. Trajectory points for the second Du Mai trajectory include those associated with the Conception Vessel or Ren Mai primary trajectory.

The third Du Mai trajectory (Figure 5.12) corresponds with the

Qiao Mai and Wei Mai, and is most beneficial in treating wind and neurological disorders. The trajectory runs bilaterally up the spine, starting approximately in the area of Bladder 23, and continues to run bilaterally over the back and top of the head, and down behind the eyes. This particular trajectory is beneficial for physical symptoms such as tremors, numbness, traumatic brain injuries, sensory issues, and other types of neurological conditions. It can also be used to treat external pathogenic factors.

Trajectory Points

Governor Vessel 16 and 20

Bladder 23

GOVERNOR VESSEL 16 WITH BLADDER 23

- Widens physical span of treatment along back and head

GOVERNOR VESSEL 20

- Pacifies wind and subdues yang (treats tremors)
- Raises yang and counters prolapse
- Benefits the head and sense organs (opens consciousness, treats numbness and loss of sensation)
- Nourishes the Sea of Marrow
- Benefits the brain and calms the spirit

POINT OF INTEREST

Once the practitioner is fluent in the theory and application of the eight extraordinary vessels, more advanced levels of the theory can be explored. For a patient who has completed at least one but ideally two iterations of the eight extraordinary vessel protocol in its entirety, the practitioner may couple the third Du Mai trajectory with either the Qiao Mai or Wei Mai. This would be most appropriate in treating conditions such as Parkinson's disease (Du Mai and Qiao Mai) or autoimmune disorders (Du Mai and Wei Mai).

The fourth trajectory begins approximately in the area of Bladder 23 and runs downward, bilaterally enveloping the sacrum, deep into the central cavity of the body into the perineum region. It is beneficial for treating all issues relating to the pelvic cavity, most notably qi stagnation. However, it is also used and proven to be beneficial for treating emotional issues manifesting as low motivation, sluggishness, and what is termed "heavy bottom," meaning difficulty in rising to take action. Heavy bottom is essentially a type of prolapse, usually in the bowel and anus region. People often describe the feeling like something is dropping or feels low, not in the right location physically. This type of syndrome can present itself as severe cases of irritable bowel, hemorrhoids, or organ prolapses.

Trajectory Points

Bladder 23 and 25

Large Intestine 11

Gallbladder 34

BLADDER 23

- Tonifies the Kidneys and nourishes essence
- Nourishes the blood and tonifies yang
- Nourishes Kidney yin
- Consolidates Kidney qi; supports Kidneys in grasping the qi
- Benefits the bones and marrow
- Regulates the water passages, resolves dampness, and benefits urination
- Benefits and warms the uterus, Ren Mai, Du Mai, and Chong Mai
- Benefits the ears and brightens the eyes
- Strengthens the lumbar region

BLADDER 25

- Supports the functions of the Large Intestine
- Transforms stagnation and alleviates pain
- Strengthens the lumbar region and legs

LARGE INTESTINE 11

- Clears heat and cools the blood
- Eliminates wind, resolves dampness, and alleviates itching
- Regulates qi, blood, and intestines
- Activates the channel and alleviates pain
- Benefits the sinews and joints

GALLBLADDER 34

- Benefits the sinews and joints
- Activates the channel and alleviates pain
- Spreads Liver qi and benefits the lateral costal region
- Clears Liver and Gallbladder damp-heat
- Harmonizes Shao Yang
- Treats wind conditions and releases exterior conditions
- Relaxes rigidity in thinking or rigidity that manifests in the body

DAI MAI

Master point: GB41

Couple point: TB5

Common trajectory points:

BL23

LR13

GB26–28

Draining Dai Mai:

LR13

GB26–28

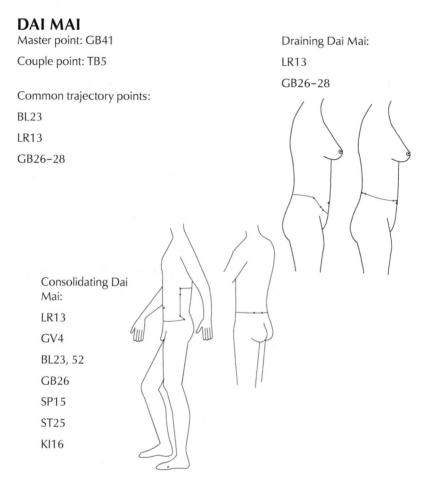

Consolidating Dai Mai:

LR13

GV4

BL23, 52

GB26

SP15

ST25

KI16

Figure 5.13 Dai Mai (Belt Vessel, Girdle Vessel)

Master Point: Gallbladder 41

Couple Point: Triple Burner 5

The Dai Mai is unique in that it (a) binds all eight extraordinary vessels together, and (b) is the only vessel of the eight extraordinary vessels to run horizontally in the body. A few of the great masters indicated the Dai Mai binds all the meridians in the body together, to include the twelve primary meridians. This makes the Dai Mai unique in its ability to transform both physical conditions and emotional afflictions.

Treating the Dai Mai is helpful with significant damp conditions (e.g., heavy bottom, feeling submerged in water, incongruence between the upper part of the body and the lower part of the body in terms of how they feel—a disconnect between the upper and the lower, or the sensation of a tight band wrapping around the mid-section). This vessel is referred to as a "regulating" vessel. In other words, treating the Dai Mai helps to regulate the body, mind, and spirit of the individual.

The Dai Mai has a primary function of storing. This can manifest physically or emotionally, or both. When it gets over-full, the excess leaks out into the other meridians in the body. Syndromes that manifest under these conditions include cysts, fibroids, edema, excess fatty tissue, stones, and pathology of the uterus, bladder, prostate, or gallbladder. It is a depository for post-natal junk. Given that the eight extraordinary vessels hold our mind stream from one life to the next, there is residual information in the Dai Mai from previous lives, which is held in the Chong Mai, along with pre- and post-natal essence. Another aspect that sets the Dai Mai apart is that it primarily holds experiences and perceptions from the current life.

Only those that can authentically describe the death bardo know exactly what happens with individual karma between lifetimes. As it relates to the eight extraordinary vessels, however, the winds and channels undergo transformation in the space between lifetimes. This process is largely based on the karma of the individual.

From a physiological viewpoint, consider dampness and wind conditions: the underlying condition is displayed via the observable manifestation of signs and symptoms. These are the primary conditions that result due to disharmony in the Dai Mai.

There are two trajectories associated with this vessel; one is generally used for consolidating while the other is for draining. If the practitioner is unclear as to what would best serve the patient, it is recommended to use the draining trajectory. It can be used to treat most conditions associated with the Dai Mai, with the exception of "leaky gut," which is mostly better served using the consolidating trajectory. The body is wise and does what is appropriate, with the MP and CP activating the channel, regardless of on- or off-trajectory points.

A common physical example of Dai Mai excess is observed in an overweight person whose fat is primarily carried around the middle jiao. This is an area where repressed emotions can be stored, especially anger and frustration. Practitioners may refer to this condition as dampness in the body, and the patient will often show other signs of dampness, such as sinus problems or fluid on lower limb joints. If heat is present, the dampness can manifest as urinary tract infections, sinus infections, diseases of the genitalia, kidney stones or gallstones, which also reflect qi stagnation. Many viruses are a result of a damp-heat condition.

Food and drugs greatly impact the Dai Mai. When used inappropriately, the substances consumed impact the functioning of the vessel. For example, all eating disorders impact the functioning of the Dai Mai, as does recreational drug use. These habits may manifest as foggy brain, poor digestive systems, lethargy, edema of the lower limbs, possible hernias, and/or prolapsed conditions, in addition to the above-mentioned conditions regarding cysts, fibroids, etc. Recreational drug use has a huge impact on the internal organs. In terms of dampness, the Gallbladder and Spleen are mostly impacted.

Emotionally and spiritually, there is a lack of motivation, co-dependency behavior, anger, frustration, resentment, inability to let go of anger, excessive worry, hypersensitivities, judgmental disposition, and often depression. These can lead to stagnation and low self-esteem.

Emotional and mental conditions most often exhibited are strong opinions (even arrogance) about the most mundane of circumstances. It is difficult for these individuals to think outside the box, be flexible in their thinking, absorb new ideas, and genuinely feel they are right about whatever it is in question. It can be difficult for them to soften the rough edges in their mannerisms.

Most patients will exhibit multiple symptoms when there is pathology in this vessel. Unlike the other vessels, those with disharmony in the Dai Mai will initially present what appears to be a mixed condition. This is because the Dai Mai is indirectly connected to all eight vessels; therefore, multiple syndromes can present themselves throughout the body. It is important to keep in mind that when the Dai Mai is activated, all eight extraordinary vessels are being peripherally impacted. In other words, the entire network of deep pathways is being awakened—touched at minimum.

The Dai Mai holds unexpressed emotions. As an individual begins to grow and experience life, ideally they evolve. The extent of evolution varies by individual. It largely depends on the health and vitality of the energetic web throughout the body, and predispositions. When the individual is not able to release emotions in a healthy manner, they become stored in the Dai Mai. Releasing emotions appropriately requires a body–mind–

spirit fluidity. The body, mind, and spirit will begin to harmonize with one another as the individual transforms and resolves stored emotions. This process can be painful either physically or emotionally. The pain is not to be perceived as something to avoid or push back. It simply means the individual is evolving and the ego wants to fight back. Giving the patient space for introspection and supporting them in obtaining a high level of self-honesty will help guide them through the process. When an individual represses growth, and neglects to listen to the inner guide, this is stored in the Dai Mai as excess—all the more reason to be mindful of our patients when treating the Dai Mai. Practitioners can never be certain what will open up in the course of treatment. It is important for the patient to have a support system in place.

Individuals with Dai Mai pathology will have tantrums. Think of a baby not able to express its emotions. The baby begins to cry as the tension is released through tears, and is soothed becoming calmer. Watch the body of a baby when crying: the middle jiao is especially tense. As the child grows, the tantrums are displayed differently because they develop the skill of language; however, if a child is not well versed at expressing through words, they can become frustrated, and this can manifest in obstinate behavior. They may begin to show physical signs around the middle jiao, even if thin and athletic. The body's ability to release tension, worry, frustration, and anger through tears is important. If a patient has difficulty crying, it would be beneficial to support the patient in cultivating the ability to cry, most often done through Liver and Gallbladder points. It is important for an individual to be able to cry, as this is the body's main avenue for releasing excess in the Dai Mai.

Unfortunately, it has become common practice to start treating a patient on either the Chong Mai or the Dai Mai. In truth, these are best left to later in the series of eight extraordinary treatments unless addressing a serious and/or acute condition. It is more beneficial for the patient to begin eight extraordinary treatments on the Wei Mai or Qiao Mai.

If wind is present, there will be ticks, spasms, tremors, and issues with balance and gait. If heat is present, there will be susceptibility to infections, cysts, bowel problems, or impaired digestion, sleep disturbances, and inappropriate sweating or orifice discharges. Body temperature is often impacted as well. If there is qi stagnation, there will be susceptibility to stones, cysts, fibroids, tumors, and uterine, ovary, or prostate problems, or general adrenal concerns.

Lastly, Dai Mai pathology can impact the functioning of Kidney yin and yang in terms of either excess (rare) or deficiency. Trajectory points are almost always used on the second and subsequent treatments of the Dai Mai. Because the Dai Mai binds the other meridians and has multiple unique qualities, specific off-trajectory points can be more beneficial with this particular vessel.

Trajectory Points
For Draining

Liver 13

Gallbladder 26–28

LIVER 13

- Harmonizes the Liver and Spleen
- Regulates the middle and lower jiao
- Fortifies the Spleen
- Spreads the Liver and regulates qi
- Treats blood issues

GALLBLADDER 26

- Resolves dampness in the lower jiao
- Regulates the Dai Mai and the uterus; regulates menstruation and stops leukorrhea
- Activates the channel and alleviates pain

GALLBLADDER 27

- Regulates the Dai Mai
- Regulates the lower jiao and transforms stagnation

GALLBLADDER 28

- Regulates the Dai Mai
- Regulates the lower jiao and transforms stagnation

For Consolidating

Liver 13

Gallbladder 26

Spleen 15

Stomach 25

Kidney 16

Bladder 23 and 52

Conception Vessel 8 (not needled)

Governor Vessel 4

LIVER 13

- Harmonizes the Liver and Spleen
- Regulates the middle and lower jiao
- Fortifies the Spleen
- Spreads the Liver and regulates qi
- Treats blood issues

GALLBLADDER 26

- Resolves dampness in the lower jiao
- Regulates the Dai Mai and the uterus; regulates menstruation and stops leukorrhea
- Activates the channel and alleviates pain

SPLEEN 15

- Tonifies the Spleen and limbs
- Regulates qi and benefits the intestines
- Resolves dampness

STOMACH 25

- Regulates the intestines
- Regulates the Spleen and Stomach
- Resolves dampness and damp-heat
- Regulates qi and blood and eliminates stagnation
- Clears heat in the Stomach and Large Intestine
- Calms the spirit and opens the mind's orifices

KIDNEY 16

- Regulates qi, alleviates pain
- Regulates and warms intestines (diarrhea/constipation, borborygmus, vomiting, leaky gut syndrome, lin syndrome)
- Treats epigastric distention, pain or cold; shan disorder
- Nourishes Kidneys and yin—most commonly used in Yin Qiao Mai
- Supports healing from trauma
- Strengthens vitality of entire system

BLADDER 23

- Tonifies the Kidneys and nourishes essence
- Nourishes the blood and tonifies yang
- Nourishes Kidney yin
- Consolidates Kidney qi; supports Kidneys in grasping the qi
- Benefits the bones and marrow

- Regulates the water passages, resolves dampness and benefits urination

- Benefits and warms the uterus, Ren Mai, Du Mai, and Chong Mai

- Benefits the ears and brightens the eyes

- Strengthens the lumbar region

BLADDER 52

- Tonifies the Kidneys and benefits the essence

- Regulates urination

- Strengthens the lumbar region

- Strengthens the will

CONCEPTION VESSEL 8 (NOT NEEDLED)

- Warms the yang and rescues collapse

- Tonifies the Spleen and original qi

- Warms and harmonizes the intestines

- Is centering

GOVERNOR VESSEL 4

- Tonifies Kidney yang and warms Ming Men

- Tonifies the original qi

- Expels cold

- Clears heat

- Tonifies and regulates the Du Mai

- Tonifies the Kidneys and essence

- Benefits the lumbar spine (treats lower back pain)

- Clears the mind

- Extinguishes interior wind

Off-Trajectory Points
GALLBLADDER 38

This is the Fire point on the Gallbladder channel, which ameliorates a timid Gallbladder, moves stagnation, and expels dampness. It helps to regulate the Gallbladder channel in general and soothes the Liver and helps alleviate "heavy bottom."

GALLBLADDER 40

This is the source point on the Gallbladder channel, which helps to regulate the meridian in a general way and support the deep pathways. It helps to modify and regulate qi, and resolves damp conditions, especially accumulations that have a downward direction or are located toward the lower part of the body.

Both of these Gallbladder points help with depression, excessive sighing, and a sense of heaviness. They help broaden a person's vision, bring clarity to what is really important in life, and help them see the bigger picture through perceptions. The Gallbladder channel is a spiritual channel and helps all the officials in the body to gain clarity and ease of movement, and creates calm so that internal work can be accomplished. It does this by helping to cultivate realistic conditions through perception (as opposed to getting caught up in the story and losing sight of reality).

SPLEEN 6

This point is associated with three yin officials (Kidney, Liver, Spleen). It tonifies qi and blood and calms the pelvic cavity in general. This point has the ability to ground a person in the midst of chaos or perceived chaos, and expels pervasive dampness in the body.

SPLEEN 7

This point helps to regulate qi and blood in the body in general and gives structure to the waterways in the body as well as the mind, to combat circular or obsessive thinking.

Both of these Spleen points aid in depression, whether chronic or acute. They help to fortify the Spleen and cultivate harmony in the Earth element in general, and aid in the calming of the Liver when upset, especially by something originating in the Gallbladder.

BLADDER 64
This is the source point in the Water element, which helps to regulate the meridian in a general way and support the deep pathways, doing whatever is appropriate. It supports the water so that jing is cared for appropriately, helps a person guide and manage resources in the body, and supports the mind.

BLADDER 66
The Water point in the Water element aids fluidity, broader perspectives, and body fluid regulation, and eases temperament both emotionally and physically. It helps to give birth to new perceptions, vision, and clarity, and helps create movement in the body in general, reducing stagnation.

BLADDER 67
The Metal point in the Water element engenders a connection between Heaven and Earth, and pre- and post-natal qi, and supports elevating the spirit (shen). It is associated with Winter, so it helps to relieve "dark clouds" and fears held deep in the body. Additionally, it helps to regulate qi and blood in the body, addresses pathology in the pelvic cavity in general, and gives a jolt to stagnant qi and/or reserves of fluid if needed. It also supports the sheng cycle in general.

All the Bladder points help to bring homeostasis to the pelvic cavity in general and are best used in combination with other points.

TRIPLE BURNER 2
This is the Water point in Triple Burner, offering balance between yin and yang, fluidity, and the ability to navigate whatever happens. It is associated with Spring, so it also helps guide perceptions, vision, and clarity, aiding the Gallbladder with digestive stagnation. It supports movement in the body, mind, and spirit, and controls the movement of fluids throughout the body.

TRIPLE BURNER 9
This is a powerful point to use when the intention is more focused on the four primaries of the eight extraordinary vessels (Chong Mai, Ren Mai, Du Mai, and Dai Mai) in terms of communication throughout the energetic web. It brings stability to the pelvic cavity specifically, helping to connect all the channels through compassionate communication, and brings balance to all officials and deep pathways.

CHAPTER 6

VERSATILE POINTS

There are several points that can be used when employing any of the eight extraordinary vessel treatments. These points are referred to as versatile points, meaning they accentuate the treatment regardless of the vessel being treated. This book highlights a total of 20 versatile points. While there are several more, these twenty are the versatile points most often used.

Versatile points have three main focus areas: communication among the channel system, movement of qi and body fluids, and harmonizing the spirit. Discernment of which versatile points to use is determined by the focus area. For example, if the practitioner has chosen to treat the Qiao Mai on the patient, and determines that accentuating the movement of body fluids would prove beneficial, a selection of points might include the MP and CP of the Qiao Mai (pairing Yin Qiao Mai with Yang Qiao Mai), and one or two versatile points that focus on the movement of body fluids. Another example is treating the Wei Mai and accentuating harmonization of the spirit. This point selection would include the MP and CP of the Wei Mai (pairing Yin Wei Mai with Yang Wei Mai), one or two trajectory points, and one or two versatile points that focus on the spirit of the individual.

The practitioner may determine that one or two or perhaps all three focus areas are important to address in one treatment. Should this be the case, it is recommended that no more than three versatile points be used in conjunction with the MP and CP of the vessel(s), and one to two trajectory points. The practitioner can mix up the selection of trajectory and versatile points as long as no more than 10–12 points in total are needled. More than 12 points within the context of an eight extraordinary vessel treatment is an exceptionally deep treatment and can cause adverse reactions such as dizziness, light-headedness, fainting, or emotional instability. Using 10–12 points in total should be determined with care and the skill of the practitioner. The purpose of point combinations is to enhance the overall treatment in one session as well as the treatment strategy or treatment plan. Point combination is critical to patient success, and therefore learning point combinations becomes critical in short- and long-term treatment planning, whether the patient is suffering from an acute or chronic condition.

MULTIPLE TRAJECTORIES

For the extraordinary vessels that have multiple trajectories (Chong Mai, Du Mai, and Dai Mai), the MP and CP are always the same, regardless of the trajectory. The body will know which trajectory is being activated based on the trajectory points selected. For example, if the fourth trajectory of the Du Mai is selected, the MP and CP are used to activate the vessel. Other points of selection could be Bladder 23, Bladder 25, and GV 1, for example. The energetic body will know the fourth trajectory of the Du Mai is the focus of treatment based on the selection of trajectory points.

Consider another example. The practitioner determines the best Du Mai treatment plan for the patient involves the second trajectory, based on patient complaints, pulse and tongue readings. Again, master and couple points are needled, with an "even technique," and trajectory points are selected (e.g., CV3 to nourish yin, CV9 to facilitate body fluids, and CV14 or CV15 to harmonize either the Heart or Pericardium). In addition to facilitating the actions associated with the corresponding CV points, the practitioner's intention in this scenario would be to activate the Du Mai for uplifting yang, providing focus, facilitating breath within the Microcosmic Orbit, and bringing balance to the patient. The patient will begin to notice a perspective that allows them to have a more positive relationship with their immediate environment.

One may argue that moving fluids, nourishing yin, and harmonizing shen can be done on the back using Governor Vessel points, and one could certainly accomplish these intentions using GV2, GV11, and GV24 or GV28. However, it is important to attend to the subtleties, and the decision to treat the primary or the secondary Du Mai trajectory rests in the discernment of the practitioner.

It is paramount to pay close attention to what the patient reports after each treatment, observing the subtleties and details, including the choice of words the patient uses.

The Versatile Points, Point by Point
KIDNEY 9

Kidney 9 tonifies the Kidneys in general and possesses a direct link to the Heart organ and Heart meridian, making it a beneficial point when supporting the patient's Kidney–Heart axis. This point in the context of an eight extraordinary vessel treatment can help maintain a sense of equilibrium that supports the patient emotionally while experiencing the effects of an eight extraordinary vessel treatment. For example, when experiencing treatment on an extraordinary vessel, there can be times and/or situations that feel more intense or unstable. KI9 can help stabilize "choppy waters" and give the water a bank to be guided by during the processing time.

KI9 is a trajectory point on the Yin Wei Mai. However, it is a beneficial "grounding point" when used as a versatile point on another extraordinary vessel. It is often used when treating the Chong Mai, for example. While not a point on the primary trajectory of the Chong Mai, KI9 is a wonderful point for fertility purposes. Other physical attributes include transforming phlegm and clearing the Heart channel, and helping to relieve pain, especially in the legs. When appropriately functioning, KI9 helps nourish a budding idea the individual may have in their professional or personal life. It gives the idea a place to formulate and be cultivated.

KIDNEY 16

Kidney 16 adds vitality to an individual. Adjacent to CV 8, it has a profound effect on the Stomach meridian and pelvic cavity. KI16 is on the Chong Mai trajectory and is used for fertility, stabilizing a Water constitution type, and treating disorders of the Stomach and abdominal pain. In general, it strengthens vitality of the entire channel network system, most especially the Kidney meridian. Regulating qi and warming the intestines, it nourishes the Kidneys, and treats Kidney yin deficiency. Like KI9, it helps maintain equilibrium in the context of an extraordinary vessel treatment, centering the patient between Heaven and Earth. This is especially important when it is used for healing trauma.

Should the patient experience fear during the course of extraordinary vessel treatments, KI16 directly addresses primordial qi and gives the patient the will to persevere.

During the course of extraordinary vessel treatments, qi should flow harmoniously in order to keep the patient moving forward, especially when addressing old wounds, trauma, and heartbreak. Stuck qi can be catastrophic most especially during an eight extraordinary vessel treatment; therefore, using KI16 while treating any of the extraordinary vessel treatments can be beneficial in ensuring adequate flow of qi in the torso and pelvic cavity.

LIVER 14

Liver 14 is one of the many "gate" points on the body. Gate points in the body are just that—gates that open, close, and connect. The areas where gate points are found are not to be left closed or open, but rather function more like valves in the heart with homeostatic and involuntary movement allowing adequate amounts of qi to flow through from one area to another. When a gate point is closed shut or left wide open, equally dangerous pathology results.

Similar to all points on the Liver meridian, LR14 helps to regulate liver qi and blood. In particular, LR14 helps to open the chest and transform phlegm. This point specifically helps the individual have a broader sense of perception and understanding of the current moment and/or situation. This can prove fruitful when treating one of the extraordinary vessels and the patient begins to have a narrower outlook. LR14 can be of particular benefit when treating the Yin Wei Mai for resolving heartbreak and reviving the spirit.

Treating extraordinary vessels creates movement; however, the movement is not always easy flowing or harmonious. Adding LR14 to the treatment adds the extra benefit of helping the patient to see "the light at the end of the tunnel," even if just beginning the treatments. Trauma victims, for example, can feel instantly overwhelmed at the thought of addressing their issues around the incident(s) that caused the trauma. LR14 aids in easy flow of qi and a greater/larger outlook when embarking upon a difficult journey. In addition, there can be a tremendous amount of processing that takes place in the patient. Processing is largely a function of the Stomach meridian, not only for food and digestion but also mental processing. LR14 is an excellent point to assist the Stomach meridian in this regard.

GALLBLADDER 20

Gallbladder 20 is a trajectory point on the Yang Qiao Mai and Yang Wei Mai. It can also be used as a versatile point on other extraordinary vessel treatments, especially when treating the Du Mai and Dai Mai. In general, this is an excellent point in addressing many wind conditions, especially those that affect the neurological system. A classic diagnosis in conventional terms would be Parkinson's disease.

It is often used to address Liver yang and Liver heat pathology. The same is true in the context of an eight extraordinary vessel treatment. Over-accumulation in the Dai Mai—from chronic frustration, for example—creates Liver heat patterns. A basic treatment might include the MP and CP of the Dai Mai, trajectory points (for draining), with versatile point GB20. This clears both wind and heat within the Dai Mai while addressing frustration, inability to let go of a situation, and/or deep resentment.

The most profound emotional effect that GB20 offers as a versatile point is its ability to help an individual make a decision and gain clarity about a situation they are having difficulty processing and/or proceeding with. It opens the mind and clears the fog.

GALLBLADDER 39

Gallbladder 39 assist with Liver wind conditions; however, it has a more profound effect on the Gallbladder channel. It assists with regulating the channel and clears heat patterns in both the Gallbladder and Liver meridians. Similar to GB20, it helps with wind conditions. What makes GB39 stand out, however, is its ability to clear heat and drain excess qi in the upper part of the body. It is extremely helpful in treating conditions such as multiple sclerosis.

In the context of an eight extraordinary vessel treatment, it has a similar effect and can be used for heat and wind conditions; however, its connections to the Bladder and Stomach meridians makes it uniquely qualified to address issues associated with these meridians, such as digestion, abdominal discomfort, swelling, neck stiffness, and difficulty with standing or lifting the limbs. When working on the Qiao Mai, for example, GB39 can be a beneficial versatile point to add to the treatment to address these types of conditions in the patient. The Qiao Mai are predominantly associated with the structure of a person both physically and spiritually. Should the practitioner decide to treat the Qiao Mai and the patient also suffers from pain in the lower limbs, especially upon standing, adding GB39 can be extremely helpful. Another example might be treating the Qiao Mai as a starting point for an iteration of the eight extraordinary vessels; if the patient suffers from chronic gastritis and fullness in the solar plexus, GB39 can help alleviate this discomfort in the context of the eight extraordinary treatment.

HEART 7

Heart 7, like LR14, is a "gate point." LI14 (Gate of Hope) functions on a physical level much like a gate opening and closing for blood and qi. It also assists in returning hope to an individual experiencing despair. HT7, while also a gate point, has more to do with the gate of the spirit. It is the place for the spirit. Precisely at HT7 is the entrance to the kingdom of the spirit. From a functional point of view, it does the obvious: regulates the Heart, transforms Heart phlegm, clears Heart fire, and tends to either the deficiency or excess of heat in the Heart and/or blood. It is a quintessential point in calming and soothing the Heart when in upset or distress. Therefore, HT7 treats all things cardiovascular including "tentacle" symptoms as a result of a cardiovascular concern.

As a gate point, HT7 is in use more than most people realize. This gate must remain fluid, opening and closing like the harmony of a seesaw in balance. Should it close shut, the individual can only see the darkness. This most often happens when a state of shock occurs. Ideally, the gate reopens in time; however, should it remain closed due to pathology, the spirit can no longer be fed or satiated. When HT7 is closed simultaneously with LI14, the individual feels total despair. This emotion is normal under certain circumstances (e.g., the death of a loved one), but in time and with guidance these gates need to reopen. Acupuncture is a great resource to assist in these circumstances.

When HT7 is used in the context of an extraordinary vessel treatment, it aids in the digestion of repressed memory that is often illuminated as a result of the eight extraordinary vessel treatment. Further, it tends to the spirit and Heart nature of the patient, allowing for a healthy integration of painful or repressed memories. Examples include using HT7 in Chong Mai treatments for fertility, especially if the patient has a history of miscarriages. In this example, HT7 tends to the Heart nature of the patient, allowing a healthy integration of memories of heartbreak so a new life can come forward. Another example is using HT7 in Yin Wei Mai treatments, again assisting with healthy integration of painful memories regarding relationships. HT7 stabilizes the spirit and creates a harmonic movement of opening and closing the gate to the Heart and the spirit of the individual; it brightens the shen.

Small Intestine Meridian

The Small Intestine meridian in the context of an eight extraordinary vessel treatment is uniquely different than any other meridian or point. This is primarily due to its ability to sort and assist in digestion, not only physically or emotionally/mentally, but spiritually. It expels heat in the Heart meridian due to shock, upset, or heartbreak. No other meridian assists a patient in "getting through the material" like the Small Intestine meridian. All Small Intestine points assist with sorting on a body–mind–spirit level; however, a few are noteworthy and therefore included in the Versatile Points section.

SMALL INTESTINE 6

Small Intestine 6 is the single most powerful point in assisting an individual in letting go of a past trauma or injury to the Heart. It nourishes on the body–mind–spirit level and supports a person who is stuck on past events, cannot fix old problems, has a chronic illness, or seems to live in difficult places emotionally and/or spiritually. It is especially good for aging people who have found themselves in nursing homes or assisted living conditions. SI6 is about nourishment.

In the context of an eight extraordinary vessel treatment, it can be combined with Du Mai, giving the patient the ability to stand up and move forward with confidence. It works well with both Qiao Mai and Wei Mai in assisting with reframing the past or present and supporting a larger perspective about a person, people, places, or circumstances and situations. In Dai Mai treatments, SI6 transforms excess and assists with clarity, vision, and seeing a way forward, releasing constraints and ties that bind the patient. SI6 revitalizes qi much like KI16, which becomes necessary when releasing the past and transforming the future.

SMALL INTESTINE 8

Small Intestine 8 is also a nourishing point, but instead of its focus on assisting in the release of the past or what is "old," it functions more as a grounding point. It brings stability to a patient, most especially in the context of an extraordinary vessel treatment. It is a solid base which can be fruitful in deeper treatments.

In general, SI8 assists in many conditions related to the upper body—the neck, shoulders, upper body muscles, arms, scalp, and head. Because of its connection to the Spleen and Stomach meridians, it aids in matters of digestion. Similarly, it supports extraordinary vessel treatments and can be especially beneficial for those with a strong Earth constitution as described in five element theory. As with several versatile points, it helps stabilize a patient emotionally when treating an extraordinary vessel. It cultivates joy and nourishes while offering a home base.

SMALL INTESTINE 10

Small Intestine 10 is helpful for "all things shoulder blade." Regardless of the conditions or injury related to the scapula or upper back, SI10 is the go-to point.

In the context of an extraordinary vessel treatment, it is a trajectory point on both the Yang Qiao Mai and Yang Wei Mai. This area, specifically the SI10 point, is where an individual initially connects with the environment. This concept can be confusing because as people walk forward, it seems logical people would meet with their environment on the Yin side or Front side of the body. However, human beings protect themselves in scenarios of danger, concern, or uncertainty, and immediately turn to the side or angle their body in a manner of protecting the Yin side. This is an interesting point. The area of the body that moves in this described "front" position is the back of the shoulder, precisely at SI10. While "carrying our burdens of life" is often associated with the Large Intestine meridian, it is the Small Intestine meridian that is doing the constant sorting of what to do next. Therefore, understanding SI10 as that meeting point between human and environment supports the theory of knowing what to do most especially in times of fear. This "knowing" is a function of the Small Intestine meridian. Another way to think of it is being faced with an image of something unpleasant and the closing of the eyes so as to not see; the body often will turn to the right or the left to face away from what is unpleasant.

As well as being a meeting point between person and environment,

SI10 is a beneficial versatile point when treating any extraordinary vessel, given its ability to help an individual accept their environment regardless of the situation or circumstances. Acceptance is a part of moving forward.

SMALL INTESTINE 11

Small Intestine 11, similar to SI10, in general is beneficial for shoulder concerns, especially the back of the shoulder and scapula. It can also be useful with conditions involving the arm and elbow. Its sorting capability is most noted when assisting with rebellious qi and supporting the digestion and dissemination of descending qi.

SI11 is a powerful point for the mental faculties of a patient, especially if they struggle to appropriately sort information involving the senses. They may suggest their minds are "clogged up" or "foggy." This is because information is being received through the senses, yet they struggle to sort the information and instead become confused. SI11 is a great point to help clean out the clutter, sort through the material, and assist the individual with dissemination of information.

In the context of an eight extraordinary vessel treatment, SI11 becomes an instrumental point in assisting the patient to sort the information that is illuminated in the course of treatment and helps prevent the patient from becoming bogged down in the information or confused by it. It is well suited to be needled with SI10 specifically with treatments involving the Yang Qiao Mai and Yang Wei Mai; it accompanies SI10. Given that the Qiao Mai and Wei Mai deal with present life issues as well as past-life issues, respectively, SI10 and SI11 help the patient sort through the material presented during the course of Qiao Mai and Wei Mai treatments. Combining SI10 and SI11 during the course of these types of treatment is especially good for individuals who have structural issues and/or concerns involving the upper part of the body—shoulders, neck, and arms specifically. This could include tremors, spasms, and pain. It is not so much about "bearing" the information and/or burdens as it is sorting through them.

SMALL INTESTINE 19

Given the location of Small Intestine 19, this point is beneficial in treating issues relating to the ear. It also makes a great heat-clearing treatment, especially in cases of ear infections, hearing loss, tinnitus, and headaches due to ear problems or local to the side of the head. While this point can be beneficial to physical ailments involving the ear, it has a strong emotional/spiritual component as well. When used in the context of an eight extraordinary vessel treatment, it helps the patient hear the spirit contained within regarding what is needed or what is next in life. If the individual is busy with too many distractions in life, it becomes difficult for them to hear what is being said by the emotional or spirit body. Sometimes they cannot hear others. It is literally a case of having so many thoughts swirling around in their head that they cannot take in any more information through the sense of hearing. SI19 helps open the orifice physically and mentally so new information can be heard, whether it be from within or from someone else.

This point can be used to support the physical structure of an individual and/or emotional discord. For example, within the context of treating the Qiao Mai for structural issues, adding SI19 supports the structure of the head and, as mentioned, the ears specifically. When used in treating the Wei Mai, it helps the patient hear the voice of the Heart spirit.

PERICARDIUM 4

Any of the Pericardium command points work well in the context of extraordinary vessel treatments, but Pericardium 4 has a unique method of calming the Heart shen, most especially when treating Chong Mai and/or Yin Wei Mai and emotional issues pertaining to the Heart are illuminated. Physically, it is a wonderful point in regulating the Heart and clearing heat; to include clearing heat in the blood, this point is uniquely poised to treat a variety of cardiovascular diseases, therefore making it a great point to include with Fire constitutions, and/or those with heart conditions. The extraordinary vessels bring forward all issues that need addressing, and when treating a patient with any type of cardiovascular disease, PC4 is recommended to mitigate negative consequences while treating iterations of the extraordinary vessels. Further, it is a quintessential point in treating emotional matters of the Heart when those issues have significantly impacted the mind and spirit.

Treating the extraordinary vessels illuminates that which needs to be resolved and in many cases this can impact the emotional stability of the patient. PC4 can mitigate any potential emotional breakdowns and address paralyzing overwhelm; for those suffering from depression, PC4 helps regain the ability to smile and leads the patient toward joy.

As the Xi Cleft point on the Pericardium meridian and gate point, it assists greatly with moving stagnation and harmonizing blood and qi on the Pericardium meridian, and blood and qi in general.

TRIPLE BURNER 5

Similar to LR14 and HT7, Triple Burner 5 is a "gate" point. This point is a gate (or valve) specific to body fluids, in particular blood, whereas LR14 functions are more specific to qi. It is the master point for Yang Wei Mai and the couple point for the Dai Mai—an especially important point all around. The functions of the Triple Burner meridian are worthy of their own chapter (Chapter 7). In terms of versatile points, TB5 is the quintessential communication point among the selected point combinations.

In addition to being specific to the flow of blood, this gate operates as an opening and closing between the internal and external. This means it has a large impact on the senses, what the senses are informing, and how that data or information is processed and, more importantly, communicated to the other officials (organs) in the body. TB5 is diplomatic and seeks harmony, and therefore its communication to other officials is compassionate. It functions on a body–mind–spirit level, making it an essential point to use often in the context of an eight extraordinary vessel treatment.

An example to illustrate the importance of using TB5 outside of the Yang Wei Mai and/or Dai Mai is treating the Yin Wei Mai for heartbreak in an individual who is closed down and refuses to get back in life and socialize with friends and family. A beneficial point combination could include the MP and CP for the Yin Wei Mai, trajectory points KI 9 and LR14, with versatile point TB5. In this context, the Yin Wei Mai is bruised at a Heart level; therefore, the intention of the practitioner would be to support the individual emotionally and help them rebuild trust and address any potential anxiousness. The trajectory points would soften the anger and support jing, and "bank" any excess water showing up as fear and/or taxing the resources (staying up late, crying, wallowing in emotional agony). The versatile point (TB5) would assist in the communication of this intention. Further, the point would support the individual with processing the internal (heartbreak, anger/resentment, taxing resources) with the external, helping them reunite with their environment, family, and friends.

It is critical for the function of serving as a gate/valve that TB5 be open in order for an individual to interact in and with their particular environment in a healthy manner. Otherwise, the person is in mental torment and daily functioning becomes extremely difficult.

SPLEEN 6

Spleen 6 is associated with the three yin officials: Kidney, Liver, and Spleen. It has the ability to ground a person in the midst of chaos, whether real or perceived. SP6 uniquely tonifies qi and blood simultaneously. It calms the pelvic cavity and expels pervasive dampness in the body. Given its ability to facilitate movement (qi and blood), resolve damp conditions, and enrich yin, similar to TB5, it is a quintessential versatile point and can be used in every extraordinary treatment. Emotionally, it is a very stabilizing point for the mind and assists in grounding a patient, helping them maintain appropriate perspective in a given situation or set of circumstances. Treating the eight extraordinary vessels can cause emotional upset in the process of moving the patient toward health and wellbeing—a cleansing action. SP6 enables the patient to remain stable throughout the process. It is especially good for someone prone to depression or a depressive state, returning them to a more positive and appropriate outlook.

Because SP6 is a junction point for Kidney, Liver, and Spleen, it treats various conditions associated with these yin officials, much the same in Traditional Chinese Medicine and/or five element treatments. In the context of using this versatile point in an extraordinary vessel treatment, the role and function of SP6 remains the same; however, it helps the individual move from a stuck or stagnate place, assisting the movement of the eight extraordinary vessel treatment process. An example might include someone who is processing trauma and continues to perseverate. Regardless of the eight extraordinary vessel being treated, SP6 supports the individual moving forward and integrating the memory in a healthy manner.

SPLEEN 21

When using Spleen 21 in the context of an extraordinary vessel treatment, this point is quickly tonified and the needle is not left inserted during the course of treatment. The primary purpose for this protocol is to reboot the system. The practitioner would either tonify the point prior to the extraordinary vessel treatment or just after when all needles have been removed. SP21 harmonizes all twelve primary channels and does this best by a tonification method. Determining the timing of the point is based on the needs of the patient. For example, if the patient at the time of treatment is exhausted, treating SP21 first can bring temporary balance to the meridians in preparation for the extraordinary treatment. If the patient is feeling well, appropriately tired after a long day of work, tonifying SP21 just after the eight extraordinary treatment can "ground" the treatment and send the patient off with an extremely harmonizing effect. As a general rule, SP21 is a nourishing point on a body–mind–spirit level and leaves the patient feeling grounded and supported. Given that it is located on the Spleen meridian, it also services blood and the cells of the body. It is often used to clear blocks, and this may prove fruitful prior to the extraordinary vessel treatment. Blocks can occur while transiting from one extraordinary vessel to the next, and therefore SP21 is a great point to use in helping the patient make the transition.

LUNG 7

Lung 7, similar to other versatile points, is also a master point and couple point in extraordinary vessels—the MP with the Ren Mai and CP with the Yin Qiao Mai. However, using LU7 as a versatile point in other extraordinary vessel treatments supports all the meridians and assists with bringing harmony to all the officials. This is important to note, because, again, during the course of treating an extraordinary vessel, the individual can become unsteady or show signs of instability. LU7, similar to SP6, can assist and support stabilizing the individual while they are moving through their emotional processes. It also helps resolve damp conditions, especially in the Lung, and is a beneficial point in treating wind, heat, and cold conditions.

From an emotional perspective, LU7 assists with managing emotions, especially when repressed memories begin to emerge, and helps to relieve tension in the upper part of the body (chest, shoulders, and neck). It nourishes yin officials and helps the patient process grief-stricken experiences that have caused paralysis by integrating the surrounding emotions. A good example is when treating the Qiao Mai and old memories regarding the death of a beloved emerge, and the individual cannot seem to fully integrate the memory of the death in a healthy manner. Adding LU7 to the treatment can be extremely beneficial in harmonizing the officials in the upper jiao and as a result supports the individual in vocalizing and processing the memory for healthy integration in the psyche. Essentially, it helps soothe the grief so it can be processed.

Combining LU7 and SP6 as versatile points in an extraordinary vessel treatment is of enormous benefit and potential. In combination, they support harmony of the meridians, stabilize mood and emotions, and give voice to troubled patients, especially those suffering from unintegrated memories of trauma. This makes both uniquely suited as versatile points in the context of an eight extraordinary vessel treatment.

CONCEPTION VESSEL 9

Conception Vessel 9 in general supports yin and increases fluids and waterway systems in the body.

CV9 is on the Ren Mai trajectory, and is beneficial in supporting patients who struggle with having good relationships. Using CV9 in the context of a Ren Mai treatment helps to facilitate flow of qi, blood, and all body fluids, especially in the gut and pelvic cavity. This makes it a critical point in treatments for fertility in male and female patients. However, it is also important as a versatile point in other eight extraordinary vessel treatments.

Given its unique ability to manage and help the body navigate body fluids throughout the body, it treats a host of conditions such as edema, abdominal pain and digestive upset, accumulation in the gut, intestinal discomfort, acid reflux or indigestion, and prolapses in the pelvic cavity (bladder, rectum, uterus). It can also help with pain in the lower back and flank sides of the back.

What makes CV9 special in extraordinary vessel treatments as a versatile point is its ability to support an individual in transition. That transition might be work-related, or in their personal life in a relationship, or in a therapeutic setting. It can also be a useful point when the practitioner stops treating a particular extraordinary vessel and starts another as part of the iteration of the eight vessels is in process. This means when finishing treatments on the Qiao Mai, for example, and starting treatments on the Wei Mai, adding CV9 helps facilitate the transition.

GOVERNOR VESSEL 4

Governor Vessel 4 operates in a multitude of ways, especially like a gate—hence its name Gate of Life, Life Gate, or Vital Gate. When it is functioning appropriately, it allows the individual to navigate life no matter the twists and turns, ups and downs, ebbs and flows of life. When it is not opening and closing appropriately, the energetic body can feel threatened. When this happens, fear becomes the modus operandi for the individual and the person will lack strength and vitality.

Similarly to CV9, GV4 helps regulate fluids in the body; therefore, when the physical pathology involves fevers or irregular temperatures (swinging hot to cold, cold to hot), GV4 assists in directing the fluids. It also can be used in acute cases of blood pressure issues. From a more emotional and/or spiritual perspective, this point can "give life back to the individual" by realigning them with their Tao, giving them the spaciousness to pursue their individual destiny, and, further, feeling more comfortable with participating in the larger or collective existence. It aids in giving the individual the richness of their life.

GV4 activates jing, lifts prolapse, and gives unconditional joy to the individual. Within the context of an eight extraordinary vessel treatment, it can give back vitality to an injured consciousness due to a type of trauma. It will enable the individual to walk a healthier Tao, bringing forth their highest qualities.

GOVERNOR VESSEL 20

Governor Vessel 20 can be used to either raise yang qi and counter prolapse or subdue yang qi, treating most "wind" conditions by benefiting the head and sense organs. Using GV20 in the regular course of treatments helps the individual stand up straight, perfectly aligned between Heaven and Earth. GV20 opens the consciousness, treats numbness and loss of sensation, nourishes the Sea of Marrow, and benefits the brain. Because of its ability to help align an individual perfectly, it calms the spirit when in upset.

When GV20 and CV9 are combined as versatile points in the context of an extraordinary vessel treatment, it assists those who have a tendency to overthink a situation, person, or memory, especially if anxiety is also present. GV20 helps clear the mind, and CV9 harmonizes the fluids helping the patient to develop a clear perspective and stop overthinking a situation negatively.

Lastly, GV20 gives perspective. Therefore, regardless of the extraordinary vessel treatment, it can give the patient appropriate perspective regarding their life and life circumstances. It does this by pulling the fragmented pieces together and aligning the puzzle to fit accordingly.

CHAPTER 7

THE ROLE OF THE TRIPLE BURNER

The Triple Burner channel is a strong communicator in the body, whether focused on the twelve primaries or the eight extraordinary vessels. It facilitates movement from a physiological perspective. More profoundly, it helps to create movement in the mind spiritually through its relationship to the Gallbladder, working with perceptions, calming the mind, and cultivating awareness.

Using Triple Burner and Gallbladder points together while a person is in a meditative posture can help raise awareness in the mind.

As with all the eight extraordinary vessel treatments—and Dai Mai treatments are no exception—individuals may experience memories and emotions as rather benign expressions. For others, it might be more difficult, and they can become emotionally unstable. Again, it is important that patients have a support system in place, as well as strong rapport and open communication with the practitioner.

Specifically, the Triple Burner is the liaison among the Chong Mai, Ren Mai, and Du Mai. These three vessels meet at two points within the Microcosmic Orbit pattern: at the perineum and in the very center of the brain, in line with the upper lip and base of the skull. We can access this central point within the head by pairing the Ren Mai and Du Mai, or indirectly when treating the Chong Mai alone. If one prefers to treat the Orbit pattern specifically, trajectory points on the Ren Mai and Du Mai or Chong Mai should consist of lower jiao points. It is best to think of the intersection of these vessels as it relates to the Microcosmic Orbit as a lotus located at the perineum. As the Orbit is accessed, it opens in the lower jiao like a lotus. The Triple Burner essentially functions as a facilitator or avenue of communication. A typical point combination would consist of the MP and CP of the Ren and Du Mai, with trajectory points either in the lower CV line or lower GV line, and a distal Triple Burner point—for example TB5, which is most common. This combination is specific to addressing the Orbit pattern alone.

Another example would be the MP and CP of the Chong Mai, Kidney points 11–16 (not all of them but perhaps one or two), and again a distal Triple Burner point. This begs the question of Triple Burner selection. A Triple Burner point should be selected based on its function to communicate. For example, should the patient also need assistance with physical issues in either of the three jiao, points can be selected accordingly. If issues of circulation are of concern, points addressing circulation of fluids throughout the three jiao can be selected. If the patient needs more attention on an emotional or mental level, TB5, 6, and 10 are good selections based on their spirit connections. However, any of the Triple Burner points 1–10 can assist on an emotional and spiritual level in addition to their service to the physical body. The most important component about the Triple Burner to note is its ability to communicate throughout not only the twelve primary meridians but also the eight extraordinary vessels.

CHAPTER 8

SPIRITUAL AXIS AND SPIRITUAL DEFICIENCY

A healthy Du Mai allows us to walk our life journey upright and with confidence. Accessing the *spiritual axis* as it relates to the Du Mai requires a specific protocol: master and couple point, and tonify a Governor Vessel point between 10 and 13, but not all of them, based on the needs of the patient. Add extra points that are located approximately one-half ACI from the GV meridian, between the GV meridian and inner Bladder meridian in the area between GV13 and GV12 on males, and GV12 and GV11 on females. These extra points are not points on a primary meridian. Ideally, a dip or valley will be felt by fingertip touch.

This protocol is used a total of three times consecutively, like the other eight extraordinary vessel treatment protocols, and is specific to accessing the spiritual axis for the purposes of treating a severe spiritual deficiency.

Use with caution, ensuring the patient is grounded, hydrated, rested, and has food in their system, specifically food remaining in their stomach, even if only a small amount. It is especially risky to treat if the person is sleep deprived and/or dehydrated.

Treating on these vessels is spiritual work even if the focus is primarily of a physical nature. The three levels of existence (body, mind, spirit) are interdependent, meaning that while the individual may be experiencing physical symptoms, the emotional and spiritual bodies are also impacted. Should the patient seek emotional and mental health through acupuncture, the physical body too will have been impacted. For example, a person who suffers from chronic depression will have depleted the physical body over time. The Kidneys and Spleen are impacted in cases of long-term depression. This, of course, drains the spiritual body, creating a spiritual deficiency.

A spiritual deficiency takes on a variety of forms, but the more common picture is a general lack of enthusiasm for positive movement and/or change, decrease in motivation especially in regard to activities that were once inspiring and passion driven, no real belief system (faith), including an atheist viewpoint (which is technically a belief system: to not believe), and an inability to achieve or accomplish projects either in a timely fashion or at all. People with a spiritual deficiency may express a generalized anger, seem cynical, or have a fatalistic point of view or perspective. Without the spiritual body being nourished, the individual can become foggy-minded and may even describe themselves as lost. They often perform day-to-day activities mostly going through the motions with no optimism or sense of purpose. Be mindful to understand these activities exist on a continuum from the subtle to the gross level, meaning there are various degrees to which an individual may be engaged with day-to-day activities. It is wise to not be overly judgmental or get into "should" conversations of what the patient may be experiencing or how they are behaving.

The Ren Mai and Du Mai share a close working relationship, interdependent on one another. The pairing of the Ren Mai and Du Mai can prove fruitful and powerful when evaluating the individual from a holistic perspective and determining the spirit of the person. When these vessels are paired, the winds and channels of the body are greatly impacted, allowing qi to move freely in an ascending and descending manner as though the person is sitting in a state of meditation but without sitting in any particular position. Naturally, it may be difficult for the individual to "hold" this meditative state, but the body will activate the channels as though the person is in a meditative posture, and the space this creates in the individual fosters healing of past karma as well as current karma. Pairing the Ren Mai and Du Mai can also be beneficial when treating conditions associated with breathing problems, cough, and shortness of breath. Pairing these vessels supports the meditative posture mentioned above by opening the chest cavity, allowing for deep breath to ascend and descend appropriately.

The practitioner would want to take into account whether the patient is exhibiting damp conditions. If this is the case, then choosing trajectory points on both the Ren Mai and Du Mai becomes important in fully supporting these extraordinary vessels with the ascending and descending of qi and breath. Treating off-trajectory that resolve damp are also beneficial in this circumstance.

i

CHAPTER 9

EIGHT EXTRAORDINARY PULSES

When we work on the eight extraordinary vessels, we can assume there will be a positive impact on the pulses. Questions that come to mind are how much change there will be, what should be expected immediately, and what should be expected later. Pulse diagnosis involving the extraordinary vessels is almost absent from any modern-day literature or case history. In fact, literature regarding eight extraordinary vessel pulse diagnosis is primarily seen through the lens of modern-day practitioners' clinical experience. In essence, until the 20th century, the extraordinary pulse picture remained a mystery to understand. What can be agreed upon is that in earlier times acupuncturists and herbalists treated the patient, and noted their pulse picture based on their discerned diagnosis. In other words, they did it backwards from how most practitioners are taught today. Today, a practitioner takes the pulses and develops a treatment plan based on this picture, along with patient complaint and their tongue, and so on. In the earliest traditions however, the pulse may or may not have been taken prior to treatment, and whatever pulse picture was noted was recorded as the pathological pulse. This method over time created a lot of confusion because specific pulses were recorded as certain conditions, and eventually the number of pulse pictures identified for a specific condition was vast. More modern-day practitioners of the eight extraordinary vessels have made valiant attempts to document what the practitioners of the past must have discovered. Over the course of time, a modern-day approach and method regarding pulse diagnosis has been developed and employed. And clinical experience has proven modern-day practitioners to be mostly correct.

Because nobody in the world knows the pulses for the eight extraordinary vessels, I have now decided to draw a diagram of this pulse diagnosis system and append an explanation after it to transmit the secrets that have remained unknown throughout the ages. (Li Shi Zhen, cited in Chase and Shima, 2010, p.161)

The hand diagram Li referred to (and developed) consist of a nine-position grid system that is essentially submerged within the current pulse-taking grid system most practitioners know and practice in the modern era. Therefore the nine-position grid system cannot necessarily be felt without penetrating through the more modern-day pulse-taking method.

It would seem that any definable pulse pattern covering multiple pulse positions might in the right circumstances reflect an extraordinary vessel pathology, and therefore be considered an extraordinary vessel pulse. (Chase and Shima, 2010, p.311)

Extraordinary meridian pulses do not occupy a single pulse position; rather, they are topological features consuming significant portions of the radial pulse (see Figure 9.1).

The Grid

	Lateral	Midline	Medial
Distal	BL	HT	LR
Middle	ST	PC	SP
Proximal	GB	LU/LI	KI

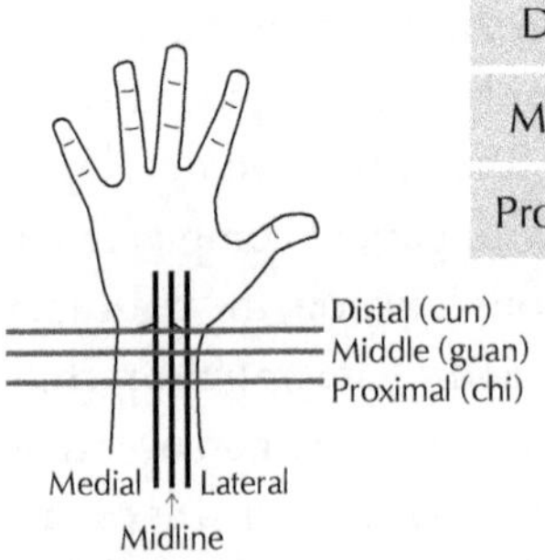

Distal (cun)
Middle (guan)
Proximal (chi)

Medial | Lateral
Midline

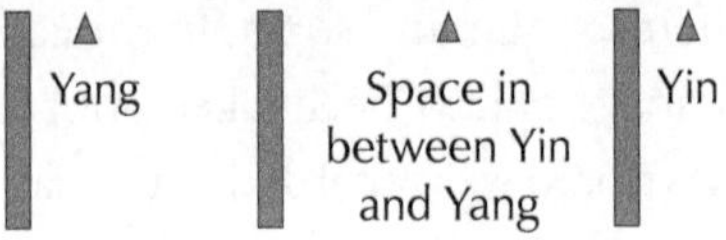

Yang — Space in between Yin and Yang — Yin

Meridian	Associated points	Meridian	Associated points
Yang Qiao Mai	MP: BL62 & CP: SI3	Du Mai	MP: SI3 & CP: BL62
Yin Qiao Mai	MP: KI6 & CP: LU7	Ren Mai	MP: LU7 & CP: KI6
Yang Wei Mai	MP: TB5 & CP: GB41	Dai Mai	MP: GB41 & CP: TB5
Yin Wei Mai	MP: PC6 & CP: SP4	Chong Mai	MP: SP4 & CP: PC6

Figure 9.1 The Pulse Grid

PULSE QUALITIES

There are various descriptors of the pulses within the nine-point grid system, and they consist of the following:

- Hard, pill-like, tapping, beating straight up and down, tense, and confined. These qualities are generally considered to be pulses of excess.

- Floating, sinking, bound, or scattered are descriptors that indicate pathogenic factors contributing to a specified condition.

Except for the Du Mai, pulse qualities can help define the exact vessel. Most of the vessels have one or more qualities that help distinguish them from the others.

For example, the Yang Wei Mai pulse passes through the Bladder, Pericardium, and Kidney positions in the hand diagram system, and yet these meridians and their representative symptoms have little bearing on Yang Wei Mai pathology.

Tapping and pill-like pulse qualities make up the vast majority of the eight extraordinary vessel theory. Tapping essentially means "tense," which is usually found on the Qiao Mai, Ren Mai, and Dai Mai pulses.

QIAO MAI

These vessels tend to run obliquely. One quality Li specified is that the Yang Qiao Mai will also have a tapping quality to it in addition to running obliquely. Additionally, if felt faint and choppy, this is indicative of wind in the Yang Qiao Mai (see Figure 9.2).

Yang Qiao Mai pathology exists when the pulse becomes tight at the Cun position and a vibration may be felt. Symptoms include cramps, mostly in the lower legs, and issues of blood circulation throughout the body, but more so in the extremities.

Yin Qiao Mai pathology exists when the pulse becomes tight at the Chi position and a vibration may be felt (see Figure 9.3). Symptoms are essentially the same as those in the Yang Qiao Mai with the exception that cramps are generally felt higher in the body (upper body), but circulation issues are the same. Both can contribute to cardiovascular issues due to their influence on the circulatory system.

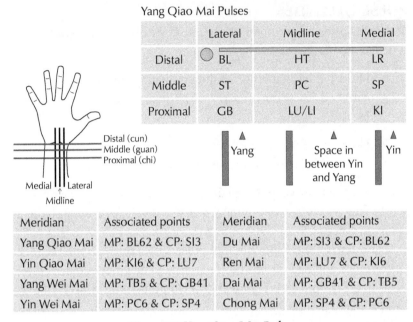

Figure 9.2 Yang Qiao Mai Pulses

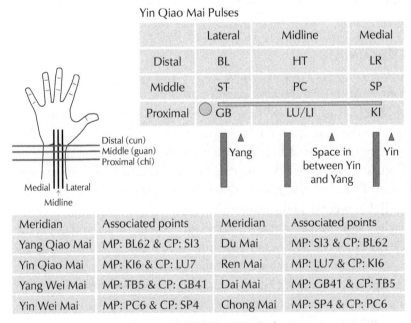

Figure 9.3 Yin Qiao Mai Pulses

WEI MAI

There is not a tremendous amount of literature specific to the Wei Mai, but the pulses appear in an oblique orientation on the wrist. Any literature regarding pulse qualities is essentially absent; therefore, it can be assumed any issues related to wei qi conditions are existent in the Wei Mai meridians and treatment would prove beneficial. In this case, patient complaints become more important in determining Wei Mai pathology, specifically the Yin Wei Mai.

Yang Wei Mai

Specific to the Yang Wei Mai pulse picture is the quality of floating. Should a practitioner feel this on the pulse (specific to this vessel), the patient will feel a sense of imbalance when standing and potentially vertigo (see Figure 9.4).

Pathology exists when pulses at the Chi position seem to roll toward the little finger or up to the Cun position and its beats are floating and excessive. Pathologies include deficient wei qi and therefore issues of heat and cold, dizziness, and disorientation (not enough wei qi to the head).

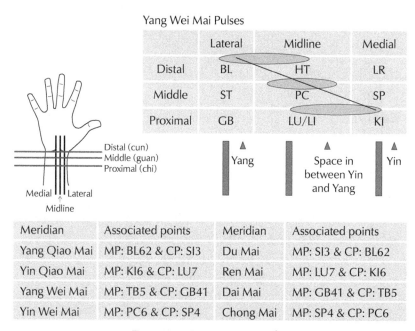

Yang Wei Mai Pulses

	Lateral	Midline	Medial
Distal	BL	HT	LR
Middle	ST	PC	SP
Proximal	GB	LU/LI	KI

Meridian	Associated points	Meridian	Associated points
Yang Qiao Mai	MP: BL62 & CP: SI3	Du Mai	MP: SI3 & CP: BL62
Yin Qiao Mai	MP: KI6 & CP: LU7	Ren Mai	MP: LU7 & CP: KI6
Yang Wei Mai	MP: TB5 & CP: GB41	Dai Mai	MP: GB41 & CP: TB5
Yin Wei Mai	MP: PC6 & CP: SP4	Chong Mai	MP: SP4 & CP: PC6

Figure 9.4 Yang Wei Mai Pulses

Yin Wei Mai

These pules are deep, large, and excessive. The patient may experience pain in the chest, a propping fullness below the hypochondrium, and heart pain. It is often described as feeling like a string of pearls. With males, there can be an excess pattern/description below the rib sides and lumbar pain, while in females there can be genital pain (sores), and the palpation will be experienced as a more "sinking" quality.

Diseases are evident when the pulses at the Chi position seem to roll toward the thumb or up to the Cun position and possess a sinking quality or excessive quality. Both sensations of the pulses are described as having a pathological component.

Pathologies include yin blood deficiency which will cause insufficient nourishment to the Heart. This may be expressed as heart/chest pain, a pinching sensation in the heart and chest area that may spread into the ribcage. Palpitations and restlessness may also be present (see Figure 9.5).

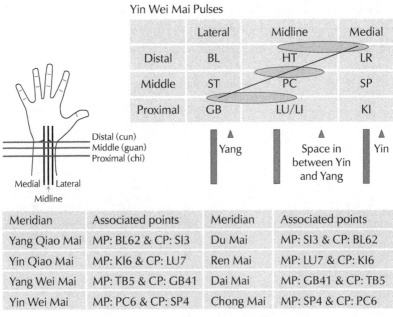

Yin Wei Mai Pulses

	Lateral	Midline	Medial
Distal	BL	HT	LR
Middle	ST	PC	SP
Proximal	GB	LU/LI	KI

Distal (cun)
Middle (guan)
Proximal (chi)

Medial | Lateral
Midline

Yang — Space in between Yin and Yang — Yin

Meridian	Associated points	Meridian	Associated points
Yang Qiao Mai	MP: BL62 & CP: SI3	Du Mai	MP: SI3 & CP: BL62
Yin Qiao Mai	MP: KI6 & CP: LU7	Ren Mai	MP: LU7 & CP: KI6
Yang Wei Mai	MP: TB5 & CP: GB41	Dai Mai	MP: GB41 & CP: TB5
Yin Wei Mai	MP: PC6 & CP: SP4	Chong Mai	MP: SP4 & CP: PC6

Figure 9.5 Yin Wei Mai Pulses

DU MAI

With a Du Mai pulse, a sure way of confirming pathology is that in all three positions a floating quality will be felt. The pulse will push straight up and down while having a floating quality to it at the same time.

Pathology can also present a wiry and "long" quality, and in all cases of pathology it is generally associated with yang deficiencies (see Figure 9.6).

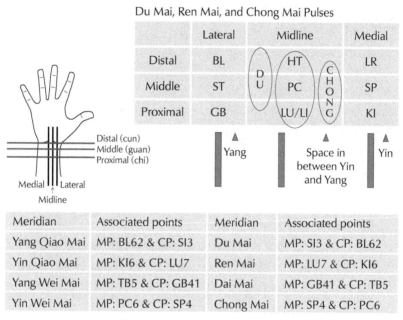

Figure 9.6 Du Mai, Ren Mai, and Chong Mai Pulses

REN MAI

Pulse qualities a practitioner may find regarding the Ren Mai include tight, fine, possibly excessive, and "long" from below up to the middle position. The quality most associated with the Ren Mai is a pill-like or pearl-like shape. Ren Mai pulses are generally felt most often in the midline position; however, these pulses extend beyond what is felt for the Chong Mai position, meaning it can be felt beyond the proximal position (see Figures 9.6, 9.7, and 9.8).

Pathology exists when the pulse is tight at the Cun position, and is thin, full, or long from the Cun to the Guan position. In general, most pathologies include a deficient cold pattern at a blood level and there is almost always a pattern of blood and/or qi stagnation.

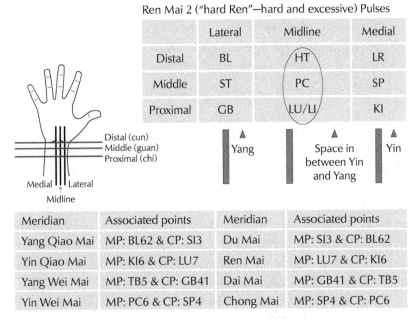

Ren Mai 1 (thin and tight/tapping in distal position) Pulses

	Lateral	Midline	Medial
Distal	BL	HT	LR
Middle	ST	PC	SP
Proximal	GB	LU/LI	KI

Yang — Space in between Yin and Yang — Yin

Meridian	Associated points	Meridian	Associated points
Yang Qiao Mai	MP: BL62 & CP: SI3	Du Mai	MP: SI3 & CP: BL62
Yin Qiao Mai	MP: KI6 & CP: LU7	Ren Mai	MP: LU7 & CP: KI6
Yang Wei Mai	MP: TB5 & CP: GB41	Dai Mai	MP: GB41 & CP: TB5
Yin Wei Mai	MP: PC6 & CP: SP4	Chong Mai	MP: SP4 & CP: PC6

Figure 9.7 Ren Mai Pulses (1)

Ren Mai 2 ("hard Ren"—hard and excessive) Pulses

	Lateral	Midline	Medial
Distal	BL	HT	LR
Middle	ST	PC	SP
Proximal	GB	LU/LI	KI

Yang — Space in between Yin and Yang — Yin

Meridian	Associated points	Meridian	Associated points
Yang Qiao Mai	MP: BL62 & CP: SI3	Du Mai	MP: SI3 & CP: BL62
Yin Qiao Mai	MP: KI6 & CP: LU7	Ren Mai	MP: LU7 & CP: KI6
Yang Wei Mai	MP: TB5 & CP: GB41	Dai Mai	MP: GB41 & CP: TB5
Yin Wei Mai	MP: PC6 & CP: SP4	Chong Mai	MP: SP4 & CP: PC6

Figure 9.8 Ren Mai Pulses (2)

CHONG MAI

The Chong Mai also can push straight up and down like the Du Mai but will have no floating qualities. It may be felt sinking and faint, and will "fill" with treatments. It is only felt in the midline position and can present as thin and/or wiry if deficient. When the vessel becomes full, it will have a hard quality to it. It too pushes straight up and down like the Du Mai (see Figure 9.6).

If one feels a "wave-like" quality on both the Du Mai and Chong Mai simultaneously, this is referred to as a "combined" pulse. It can be difficult to discern between the Chong Mai and Du Mai pulses. One way to discern is to take the pulses on both sides of the wrist. If the same quality is found on both wrists, it is a combined pulse. Chong Mai and Du Mai pulses can be felt on just one wrist, but are not necessarily felt on both wrists. In other words, a practitioner can make a judgment on the eight extraordinary vessels based on one wrist unless listening for the combined pulse.

Diseases are evident when all three positions are firm and uninterrupted; the pulse will be wiry and full (excessive) or wiry and deficient. Pathologies include pain in the abdomen as qi is not harmonic in this region of the body and/or stagnant.

DAI MAI

Pulse quality on the Dai Mai is generally a tapping/tense sensation when in disharmony. This pulse is felt in the left and right positions (superficial as well as deep simultaneously). The pulse usually has a "hard" feeling to it, similar to the hardness one feels with the Chong Mai. However, unlike the Chong Mai, the Dai Mai will have a bouncing quality (see Figure 9.9).

Disease is evident when the pulse becomes tight at the Guan position with beats that vibrate right to left (back and forth). Pathologies include inappropriate leakage in the pelvic cavity, and pain in the navel or navel area, and lower abdomen.

Dai Mai Pulses

	Lateral	Midline	Medial
Distal	BL	HT	LR
Middle	⊙ ST	PC	SP
Proximal	GB	LU/LI	KI

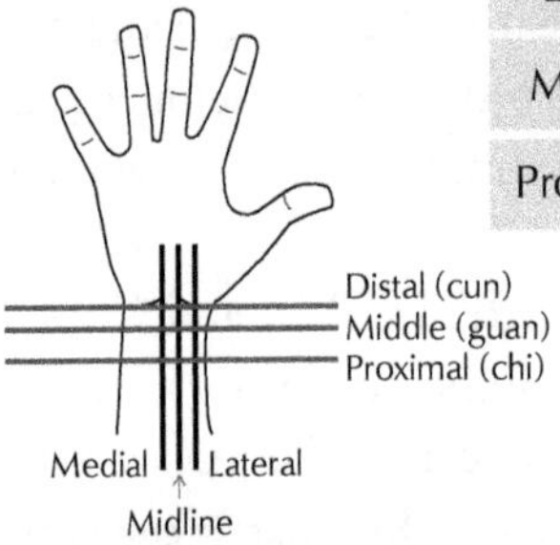

Distal (cun)
Middle (guan)
Proximal (chi)

Medial | Lateral
Midline

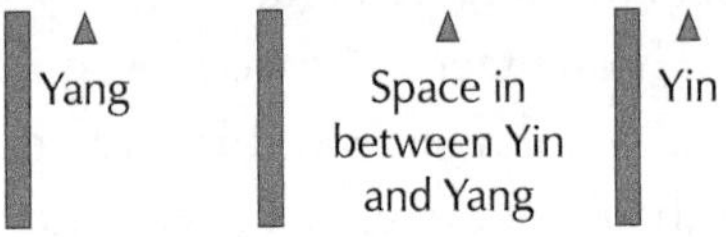

▲ Yang

▲ Space in between Yin and Yang

▲ Yin

Meridian	Associated points	Meridian	Associated points
Yang Qiao Mai	MP: BL62 & CP: SI3	Du Mai	MP: SI3 & CP: BL62
Yin Qiao Mai	MP: KI6 & CP: LU7	Ren Mai	MP: LU7 & CP: KI6
Yang Wei Mai	MP: TB5 & CP: GB41	Dai Mai	MP: GB41 & CP: TB5
Yin Wei Mai	MP: PC6 & CP: SP4	Chong Mai	MP: SP4 & CP: PC6

Figure 9.9 Dai Mai Pulses

CHAPTER 10

THE PSYCHOLOGY
OF EMOTION

The craving for pleasure or wanting to avert suffering is the result of feelings. As long as we are human, we will experience emotions. The purpose of treating the eight extraordinary vessels is to integrate healthy emotions with a healthy body and mind. These vessels assists in the integration of developing wisdom, which leads to appropriate response, appropriate expression, and the fluidity of one to the other. When treated, the eight extraordinary vessels release memories, whether from the current lifetime or a previous lifetime. For this reason, there is a particular strategy in working with the vessels. The intention is to help the person release the memories in a way that allows them to work through the process with minimal psychological consequences. Treating the eight extraordinary vessels can help a person through the lowest of times, but it can also cause added stress and risk if not done properly by the practitioner.

There is no scientific consensus regarding a definition of "emotions," or how many emotions actually exist among humans. Most studies suggest anywhere from four or five basic emotions to as many as 54. These are only basic emotions. There are many variations within the basic emotions. For example, sadness and anger both have degrees or levels of sadness or anger. The more common emotions include happiness, enjoyment, sadness, disgust, fear, surprise, anger, and contempt, with variations in each of these categories.

With the intention of using an extraordinary vessel to treat emotional issues, a concise method is to understand the original platform from which emotions come forward in the individual, the initial response, and then the actual expression of the emotion. This process can be experienced in as little as one second or as long as one minute. Or the individual may become stagnated in the process while "sorting" the event (conversation, circumstance, location, etc.) emotionally.

An individual's constitution plays a pivotal role in the development of knowledge and wisdom, as well as how they will respond or react to any given situation, and the emotion that is expressed as a result of the response and/or reaction. This is one reason why understanding even a basic level of five element theory is beneficial. All phenomena come from the five elements; therefore, before explaining the origination of emotion and its eventual expression, it is beneficial to understand how the five elements respond to each other in an individual.

The five elements are Water, Wood, Fire, Earth, and Metal. In Tibetan Medicine and philosophy, they are Water, Air, Fire, Earth, and Space. It is not necessarily important to think of these two classifications differently, only to keep both in mind when diagnosing a patient. Without going too deeply into five element theory, an important factor to remember is the Shen cycle; Water gives to Wood, which gives to Fire, which gives to Earth, which gives to Metal, which gives to Water, and so on, over and over. People fluctuate and ebb and flow from one element to the next throughout the day: laughing, listening, raising voices, being quiet, sitting, standing, and communicating each day. How a person is able to ebb and flow in and out of the emotions which are originated in the five elements depends on what information the senses bring to the person: smell, taste, hearing, seeing, touch. While all five elements are a part of the process, there are one or two elements or the dynamic between two or more elements that influence this process. For example, an individual who has a dominant Fire element will process information differently from someone who has a dominant Metal element. Again, without going into too much detail regarding five element theory, it is important to note that constitutional nature plays a role in the emotions.

The other important cycle within five element theory is the Ko cycle, which suggests a particular type and kind of communication among the elements. With the Ko cycle, Water influences Fire, Fire influences Metal, Metal influences Wood, Wood influences Earth, and Earth influences Water. The focus of this influence is more about the dynamic and communication between the elements, meaning two or more elements are equally in motion in that particular instance. This is the more common dynamic when it comes to expressing the emotions.

These cycles and the health of them in the individual contribute to the emotional knowledge and wisdom, also known in some circles as the emotional quotient (EQ) of a person. EQ is described as a person's ability to process and respond and/or react to various situations, people, and circumstances that occur on an individual life trajectory. The intelligence quotient (IQ) and EQ of an individual can be on a par with one another, or there can be a large gap in between. Because a person has a "high" IQ does not automatically indicate they manage their emotional lives with the same level of discipline or knowledge. In fact, some of the smartest people in the world struggle with interpersonal relationships and expressing appropriate emotions and/or responses to external events. This gap between IQ and EQ can be expressed as a stoicism that is pathological in its nature.

This IQ/EQ gap may have a variety of causes: childhood development, trauma, birth defects, birth order, or genetics, for example. In growth development stages, the EQ can stagnate at any point, leaving the individual at a particular age emotionally, regardless of chronological age. Left untreated or uncultivated, the individual grows into an adult with a "low" EQ. Childhood trauma (or the perception of trauma) plays a critical role in growth development. A loving and supportive childhood has the same level of influence on the individual emotionally. Further, how a child sees and perceives the emotions of their parents leaves a lifelong imprint.

To summarize, the five elements play a role in the emotions. Dominant elements in an individual play a role in the expression of the emotions. Combined with the EQ, these elemental factors establish emotional responses for the individual, and their ability to sort sensory information. Once the mental process and sorting take place, the reaction is one of attraction, aversion, or neutral. Within each category there are primary emotions that are the most common responses and reactions.

REACTION VERSUS RESPONSE

A reaction to a given person, communication, or set of circumstances is a form of response. The primary difference between response and reaction is the space in between the event and the response to the event. When a person has an immediate reaction to the event, they are simply reacting to the event. There is no processing actually occurring, only reacting to the stimulus in front of them. When an individual takes a pause or a moment to contemplate the stimulus, a response follows. Reactions and responses are consistently occurring from one moment to the next. In one moment, a reaction occurs while in another a response occurs. For example, a healthy reaction is the removal of a hand when it touches something hot. An example of an unhealthy reaction occurs when an individual has a violent outburst in response to a mundane event or communication. Instead of taking the pause and appropriately processing the stimulus, the individual immediately overreacts. It is human nature to experience the fluidity of reaction versus response. The higher the EQ, the more able the individual is to discern which is more worthy in the moment—a reaction or a response.

ATTRACTION, AVERSION, OR NEUTRAL

- The category of *attraction* means what is being communicated through one or more of the senses is appealing, accepting, interesting, and/or arousing curiosity.

- The category of *aversion* means what is being communicated through the senses is not appealing, not accepting, not of interest, and/or not provoking curiosity.

- The category of *neutral* simply means there is no response; the senses are not attracted or experiencing any aversion. There is no opinion or immediate acceptance of the information the senses are gathering.

Attraction, aversion, or the position of neutral happen almost instantly and often involuntarily. By definition, they are reactions. However, an individual can move from one to the other quickly, depending on the gathering of more information or if a better understanding takes place in the moment. A simple example is trying a new dish in a restaurant and upon first glance having an aversion. However, trying the new dish and discovering it to be quite tasty then shifts aversion to attraction. This fluidity happens throughout the day, every day, in every person.

THE PROCESS

The extraordinary vessels assist in aligning the individual on a body–mind–spirit level, addressing not only issues of the current life but also those of previous lives. As a result, memories are released which can manifest into physical, mental, spiritual, or emotional issues. Because extraordinary vessel treatments are profound in their workings and functions, emotions are in play the majority of the time. Therefore, learning and understanding where emotions originate and manifest become important not only to the patient's growth and learning but also to that of the practitioner.

Figure 10.1 demonstrates the process with the common expressions of emotions. As the practitioner treats the extraordinary vessels on a patient, this diagram can be useful in determining underlying emotional patterns. For example, if the patient expresses the emotion of sadness (they may use the word "depression"), that would indicate an aversion to the stimulus and/or event or set of life circumstances. How best to treat the aversion depends on:

1. Dominant elements within the person's constitution.

2. The suspected status of the patient's EQ.

3. Symptoms the patient is reporting.

Yin/yang and the development of the eight extraordinary vessels				
Constitutional nature/five elements				
Fire	Earth	Metal	Water	Wood
Level of development of knowledge and wisdom/emotional quotient (EQ)				

Reaction/response to stimulus–event

Attraction	Aversion	Neutral
Joy	Anger/frustration	Empathy
Happiness	Disgust	Understanding
Like/love	Contempt	Acceptance
Content	Dislike	Mourning/grief*
Surprise	Fear	
Curiosity	Sadness	

* To grieve is a process of accepting; this can take a long time depending on the circumstances

Figure 10.1 Table of Emotional Expressions

When treating a patient specifically for an emotional issue, the practitioner would follow the protocol guidelines stated in Chapter 4. Consider the three questions mentioned above, and then use this information to make a decision regarding trajectory points and versatile points. Because emotions can be expressed regardless of the extraordinary vessel being treated, trajectory points and versatile points on the extraordinary vessel are the critical component in treating the emotion(s).

EAST/WEST

Conventional medicine uses labels to identify the emotions in pathology. For example, rapid cycling between extreme joy and extreme sadness might be labeled bipolar disorder, which has variations, meaning it manifests differently in people. As a general rule, it is mostly managed with medication. Depending on the severity of the pathology, the patient may be best served using both medication and acupuncture. In milder cases, acupuncture alone may be enough. There can be multiple approaches in terms of method of treatment.

While depression has been common throughout human existence, it has become better understood with multiple studies into its causes and cures. Depression as a psychological condition operates on a continuum from mild states of depression (lows) to extreme states of depression potentially leading one to suicidal ideation. Unfortunately, suicide is more common than many realize. Current suicide rates are the highest they have been since documentation began. Most adults can work through mild depression at some point, becoming more familiar with their individual moods and how they show up in their daily life. For some, it can be beneficial to take a mild antidepressant, especially during seasonal shifts or harder emotional phases of life (e.g., following the death of a loved one). These pharmaceuticals are best when used to help the person "over the bump," but should not become long-term crutches. Many mild forms of depression can be easily managed without medication as long as the patient is receiving consistent acupuncture treatments.

When a person's moods have reached more extreme levels, and they have started contemplating suicide, they have also reached a point of no longer caring about the suffering in the world. This may sound harsh, but the reality is that the mind has entered a fatalistic viewpoint and is no longer functioning in a reality with appropriate perception. This person often has an extreme dislike of the self and is quite possibly in a state of complete breakdown.

There are approximately 150 diagnoses of mental disorders in the *Diagnostic and Statistical Manual of Mental Disorders* (DSM-5 (fifth edition)).[1] What is important for the practitioner to understand is the translation between the language of conventional diagnosis and holistic or Eastern diagnosis. Further, treating on the extraordinary vessels can manifest a swing of emotions in the patient. Again, this is why trajectory and versatile points are especially important when treating the emotions. The idea is to treat and heal the pathology that resides in the extraordinary vessel, and using specific trajectory and versatile points assists with mitigating potential surges of emotions. Think of the work as stabilizing the pendulum that swings back and forth with varying degrees of emotion. The practitioner sets the intention of supporting a homeostatic movement of yin and yang, and the space in between.

Emotions are the expression of the response and/or reaction as outlined in Figure 10.1. An example of emotional swings while treating the extraordinary vessels on a patient might appear something like this: A patient comes to you for chronic joint pain that cannot be explained by conventional methods such as imaging and/or blood work. The patient does not want to take pharmaceuticals on a regular basis to manage the pain and makes an acupuncture appointment hoping to address the issue with holistic methods. After a few treatments, the pain lessens but never fully goes away (i.e., the patient does not fully recover). Based on other symptoms, you determine the patient would benefit from an extraordinary vessel treatment and you begin with pairing Yin Qiao Mai with Yang Qiao Mai to address the structure of the patient (muscles, joints, bone, tendons, etc.). In addition, you determine the patient to have a constitution that most resembles the Fire element or having a strong affinity to the Fire element. Lastly, you have the understanding that the extraordinary vessel treatment would assist the patient in releasing trauma that may be stored in the physical body.

Generally speaking, the degree of opening Pandora's box is unknown. A suggestion for the beginner is to select a couple of trajectory points that provide perception, appropriate decision making, and the ability to move

---

1   American Psychiatric Association (2013) *Diagnostic and Statistical Manual of Mental Disorders* (fifth edition). Washington, DC: APA.

forward in life (Gallbladder points come to mind). In order to mitigate any potential surges of emotions that might prevent the patient from maintaining emotional stability, versatile points on the Heart meridian can prove useful. If you determine the patient to have more of a Wood constitution, versatile points on the Liver meridian may prove useful in harmonizing Liver qi and/or Liver blood, for example.

The emotional stability and innate constitutional nature play a role in which versatile points might be best suited within the context of the extraordinary treatment. Many patients will do well with the Qiao Mai points alone, while others will need more points needled, depending on the intention of the practitioner.

After three successful treatments on the Yin Qiao Mai with Yang Qiao Mai, you determine that the patient is doing better, pain has improved, and the patient describes a sense of feeling lighter regarding the burdens they are carrying. This is the ideal scenario. However, should the patient report what appears to be an adverse response after the first or second Qiao Mai treatment, the trajectory and versatile points become necessary to mitigate the surge of emotion which can take on the expression of anger, jealousy, and/or resentment. Therefore, using points to balance qi and blood and stabilizing the constitution are critical. HT7 can be a great point for stabilizing the emotions regardless of constitution; points on the Kidney and Stomach meridians help the individual digest and integrate information and memories, moving them from rough waters to a safe and stable harbor. Knowing the points and what they do in the body is not only critical to the health and wellbeing of the patient, but critical to the success of the practitioner and their intentions with treatment.

EMPLOYING THE EIGHT EXTRAORDINARY VESSELS TO TREAT THE EMOTIONS

Identifying when and how to employ the eight extraordinary vessels for treatment of the emotions can be difficult for the beginner (see Table 10.1). Most especially when starting a new patient for emotional concerns, it is best to start Qiao Mai treatments. The practitioner can either pair these vessels or do them one at a time, depending on the emotional stability of the patient and if there are any accompanying physical symptoms, especially pain. Needle action when using the eight extraordinary vessel theory should always be done slowly, not rushed, and gently. Ideally, there is no thrusting or vibrating of the needles except in rare circumstances and only then by an advanced practitioner.

After treating the Qiao Mai, the practitioner would treat the Yin Qiao Mai and the Yang Qiao Mai, individually or as a pair. Treating the Qiao Mai and Wei Mai first enables a solid foundation to be in place prior to employing the primary vessels. An analogy would be to build a solid foundation, framing for structure, and a roof before the inner build of the home. It is impossible to create rooms complete with drywall and paint without having built the foundation, framing, and roof first. It is much the same when employing the eight extraordinary vessels, most especially when addressing the emotions; it is best to treat the structure of the person prior to employing the deeper troves of the primaries.

Table 10.1 Eight Extraordinary Vessel Table of Emotion Pathology Identification

Yin Qiao Mai	Yang Qiao Mai	Yin Wei Mai	Yang Wei Mai
nightmares unable to enjoy life alcohol abuse insomnia sadness depression deep fear anxiousness	depression overwhelmed restlessness secrets insomnia nervous tension haunted by the past	lack of trust pensiveness obsessed emotionally torn apprehension heartache phobias anxiousness	forgetful confused indecisive lack of trust inaction focused on the past obsessive little or no willpower little or no self-control
Chong Mai	**Ren Mai**	**Du Mai**	**Dai Mai**
anger depression fear worry intergenerational imprinting obsessive-compulsive negative thinking and/or fatalistic easily addicted to substances projects internal thoughts upon others	grief fear anxiousness sadness depression inappropriate laughter extremely introverted internalizes emotions easily addicted to substances ridden with phobias	lacks ambition lacks determination cannot fully participate in life day-to-day activities are difficult over-controlling afraid of letting go still and/or rigid thinking emotionally/mentally inflexible likes to argue/debate mood swings insomnia	indecisive hard to commit frustrated/judgmental hypersensitive snaps to judgment vengeful and/or vindictive bitter and domineering often selfish overly opinionated/likes to be right rigid with negative thoughts

CASE STUDY 1

The patient is a 38-year-old female, married with one child who is three years old. She has a long history of childhood trauma and has been in therapy for several years. The patient described herself as doing pretty well until she had her son and began to suffer from post-partum depression. Her childhood issues resurfaced soon after becoming a parent. The patient's healthcare team prescribed various antidepressant medications that came with unwanted side effects such as severe neck tension which led to headaches and discomfort in her neck and shoulders. The psychiatrist changed her medication, and although the change seemed to help, the neck and shoulder tension continued. Her cognitive therapist referred her to acupuncture to address the tension and support her emotional needs, believing therapy and acupuncture in tandem would be of great benefit.

Pulse pictures indicated tight/taut pulses in general with Liver and Gallbladder meridians thread. Eight extraordinary pulses indicated Ren Mai pathology. Tongue presentation was red with a greasy and yellowish coat.

The patient has been in acupuncture treatments for approximately six weeks, receiving seven treatments. The first six treatments focused on providing pain relief using TCM methods and supporting her Earth element constitutionally with Stomach and Spleen command points. Further, coaching on self-talk and internal dialogue was initiated. Her tendency included a hyper-focus on the negative and what was going wrong versus being able to see the small measurements of "success" or improvement. Dominant elements that have the strongest dynamic include the Wood and Fire elements (slightest agitation leads to a quick and violent reaction of heated anger); however, her true constitutional nature is that of the Water element.

At treatment 7, the Qiao Mai were employed to support her physical structure (tendons, connective tissue, and bone) as well as her emotional structure (keeping events in proper perspective, balancing her emotions with equilibrium, and addressing her hypersensitive feelings). The patient described herself as experiencing the slightest critical comment as an attack on her ability to perform, whether the performance was professional (work-related) or personal (at home, as a wife, or as a mother). The quick upward-rising yang was leaving her yin very depleted, resulting in significant imbalances in yin and yang qi. Yang qi would rise too quickly with ferocity, leaving her exhausted after a fit of anger. Therefore, pairing the Qiao Mai to bring balance to the yin and to the yang simultaneously was another factor in the treatment strategy.

The first Qiao Mai treatment consisted of pairing the vessels, using off-trajectory point LR3 for hormonal balance and smooth flow of qi, versatile point LR14 for inspiration and hope, off-trajectory point CV12 for digestion of thoughts and emotions and to support Stomach qi, and versatile point GV20 for Heaven and Earth alignment, raising yang appropriately, giving her the ability to stand up and move forward despite her feelings of overwhelm, without bursting into a fit of rage. After this treatment, the patient was able to have six straight days without fighting with her husband—a much-welcomed improvement. Although it was a difficult week emotionally, she managed not to have any violent reactions and outbursts with her husband. Her neck and upper back felt relaxed for several days. The patient had a difficult time seeing the progress she had made, being hyperfocused on the seventh day when she became increasingly irritated. During the coaching portion of the treatment, the success of six days of maintaining enough balance and equilibrium to avoid a violent outburst needed to be acknowledged. Once it was pointed out, the patient was receptive, although her fatalistic outlook remained. With more coaching, she was able to acknowledge that success and improvement may come in small steps. Further, a lot of small steps leads to one stable path of health.

Future treatments will consists of multiple treatments on the Qiao Mai (paired) before employing the Wei Mai, and eventually a complete iteration of the primary vessels. The first few Qiao Mai treatments will incorporate trajectory points such as KI8 for helping her have faith in herself and begin to shift self-image issues, as well as other Kidney and Stomach points on the trajectory for digestion of memories, safely integrating them into the tapestry of her life. Healthy Qiao Mai will set the stage and create a solid platform for the continuation of the extraordinary vessel treatments, leading the patient to a healthier, more balanced life, experiencing appropriate emotions. Realistically, this process could take a year or more of consistent treatments; therefore, it is important for both patient and practitioner to have patience with the process and not rush outcomes. This patient is likely to have multiple setbacks during the course of long-term treatment, so it is important to embark upon a treatment strategy of steadiness and stability.

CASE STUDY 2

The patient is a 50-year-old male, single, and has no children of his own. His girlfriend has four children, but he does not have a close relationship with them and only sees his girlfriend occasionally. Upon meeting his girlfriend, who became interested in acupuncture, it became apparent they were only friends. However, the patient refers to her as his girlfriend. After two treatments, the patient's girlfriend did not return to acupuncture.

The patient owns and operates a small farm that he enjoys. Additionally, he works for a large utility company as a supervisor. An animal lover, he has two dogs and two cats, and enjoys being outside and using his hands. When he first started acupuncture, he had recently given up sugar and was becoming more conscientious about his diet. He drinks a lot of water and does not consume alcohol. He is of average height, and while he is not obese, tends to carry more weight than he would prefer.

The patient's initial interest in acupuncture included complementing his cognitive therapy work with a nearby therapist in order to help him with his interpersonal relationships, both personally and professionally. He indicated that he did not feel balanced and believed this to be interfering with his ability to trust others and have meaningful relationships. At the intake session, the patient appeared sad and indicated that he been feeling "depressed." When asked about suicidal ideation, he indicated he did not intend to take his own life but could understand why others ultimately made that decision. The idea of spending his life consistently at a low point seemed overwhelming. His only physical complaint included pain and swelling in his right knee and mild allergies. He reported experiencing a disturbance with his sleep occasionally and believed that to be a result of anxiety from the work day. Lastly, the patient had been diagnosed with Lyme disease.

His pulses were erratic at the first treatment session. After two clearing treatments, his pulses became less erratic, no blocks were present, and his Kidney pulse was the lowest of the 12 meridians. Eight extraordinary pulses indicated Yin Wei Mai pathology. His tongue presentation indicated heat in the Heart channel with mild Spleen qi deficiency.

After the first few treatments which were focused on clearing and constitutional support, the Qiao Mai were employed to support his physical and emotional structure. A total of six Qiao Mai were treated, consecutively starting with Yang Qiao Mai. After these treatments, the patient expressed feeling significantly better, balanced, and that he was gaining a larger perspective about his job and the people that he supervises. He continues his therapy sessions as well. At treatment number 12, he reported working on his farmhouse, buying new equipment for the land and appliances for his home, and that he had found and adopted two kittens.

Witnessing this patient having the ability to smile, laugh, and make a joke in the timeframe of six months was astonishing, given his disposition at the first treatment session. During the Qiao Mai treatments, a combination of trajectory, off-trajectory, and versatile points was used, including trajectory points such as BL59 and 61 for regulating qi, dispelling wind, and nourishing the connective tissues; KI2 and 8 for supporting Kidney qi and clearing heat; off-trajectory points BL41, 42, and 66, again for nourishing the connective tissues, addressing panic in the upper jiao, and calming the spirit; TB2 and CV9 for harmonizing water passages; LI5 for relaxing the chest; and versatile points HT7 for calming the Heart shen, GV4 and 20 for lifting yang, and KI9 for supporting matters of the Heart.

Future treatments will include the Wei Mai, consecutively, and eventually all four primary vessels in the order of Chong Mai, Ren Mai, Du Mai, and Dai Mai. This treatment strategy is a long-term strategy steered by what the patient reports, any potential illnesses that present themselves, and pulse and tongue presentations. Lastly, a Chinese herb was recommended at treatment number 11 to assists in expelling heat and supporting Kidney qi.

CHAPTER 11

CLINICAL APPLICATIONS SPECIFIC TO CONCEPTION AND FERTILITY

Historically, the Chong Mai has been the more common and favored vessel of the eight extraordinary vessel system. While the Chong Mai certainly plays a pivotal role in both conception and pregnancy sustainment, the precise strategy to employ depends on a few key factors.

- Is the patient male or female?

- What is the constitutional nature of the patient? Which of the five elements do they present more dominantly?

- Is the patient currently involved with a fertility clinic and undergoing conventional treatment, or are they considering acupuncture prior to conventional measures?

- Can the patient provide laboratory results and/or semen analysis?

- What is the age and lifestyle of the patient, medical history, and medications (past and current)?

There can be other concerns to take into consideration, but these five questions are critical to answer prior to employing the eight extraordinary vessel theory specifically for fertility purposes. The practitioner will want to take into consideration the current emotional and mental disposition of the patient given that the extraordinary vessels have an impact on the emotional and spiritual axis in the body.

MALE FERTILITY

Male fertility is generally, but not always, an issue identified through semen analysis. The practitioner will want to become familiar with how best to read and interpret the analysis. In most cases, in addition to acupuncture the patient will benefit from Chinese herbs, and there are several good formulas for this purpose. There are no absolutes, and therefore there is no one way of employment of the extraordinary vessel theory—meaning there is no one answer on how best to approach fertility issues. Generally speaking, for males, starting on the Chong Mai is a good rule of thumb if the patient is healthy, not on a lot of medication (if any), and active. If the patient is not active, coaching is necessary to help the patient become more active in order to generate adequate flow of blood and qi. It is not uncommon for males to develop blood stagnation in the testicles, so addressing blood stagnation will become important in the overall strategy. The practitioner can use off-trajectory points on the Spleen meridian paired with the Chong Mai to support this condition. Often, off-trajectory Liver meridian points can also be beneficial. A typical treatment might be: Chong Mai (MP and CP—remember with males the MP is on the left and the CP is on the right), KI13, CV4, LR9, and a Spleen point (1–8 depending on pulse, tongue, and presenting symptoms). Essentially, you want to expel damp and move blood. This is one of many options and an example of how to combine points with the Chong Mai in treating male fertility issues. While the Chong Mai needles would stay inserted for 20–30 minutes, the off-trajectory needles would be removed after approximately 10–15 minutes. The off-trajectory needles can go in at the beginning of the treatment or they can be inserted for the last 15–20 minutes of the treatment. In either case, the tonification action for the on- and off-trajectory points is used, while the Chong Mai MP and CP are inserted using an "even technique."

In summary, ideally the practitioner includes Liver and Spleen points if/when using Chong Mai for male fertility. Low CV points such as CV2–6 are also greatly beneficial. Again, there are a number of ways to approach the patient, and the five key questions above are important to take into consideration. A lot of factors can be involved with male infertility, and it can take as long as a year before acupuncture and Chinese herbs enhance semen deficiencies. Please see the list of on- and off-trajectory points in Chapter 5 for many other point options.

FEMALE FERTILITY

Female fertility is usually more complicated. History is important to take into consideration. Does the patient have a history of issues conceiving, or does the patient have a history of issues sustaining pregnancy (i.e., miscarriages)? How to go about treatment is determined by what the goals are, given the patient's situation. For example, if the patient can conceive under more normal conditions, but has a pattern of miscarriage by 12 weeks, the strategy will be slightly different from the strategy for a patient who can carry full-term but has a difficult time with conception.

For conceiving purposes, the treatment strategy can be pairing the Ren Mai with the Chong Mai. This is not a normal pairing outside the strategy of female fertility. In the beginning, it is safer to use these two vessels only with minimal trajectory points. Off-trajectory points are usually not needed unless the patient has not conceived after 4–6 treatments. If after several treatments of activating the Ren Mai paired with Chong Mai and a few trajectory points, the patient is still not pregnant, off-trajectory points can be added. The timing of the treatments with the patient's menstrual and ovulation cycle is vital to the overall strategy as well.

A typical treatment strategy would be pairing Ren Mai and Chong Mai as noted above and adding KI13, CV4, and moxa on the lower abdomen. A variation of this treatment is ideal for approximately 3–4 treatments. Eight extraordinary vessels points are needled "even," while the trajectory points are tonified. Ideally, the first three treatments would be done once a week leading up to ovulation. If the patient becomes pregnant, the practitioner should stop the eight extraordinary vessel treatment and return to points supporting Spleen, Liver, Kidney, and Conception Vessel protocols for sustaining pregnancy. If the patient does not become pregnant, the practitioner should repeat or do a similar treatment strategy beginning right after the patient's menstrual cycle, and again leading up to ovulation. Should the patient not become pregnant after these two attempts, the practitioner can add in specific fertility points such as LR9, SP10, KI12–16, low CV points, and a significant amount of moxa unless the patient has a more severe heat pattern (which could be part of the issue). See fertility points outlined in Chapter 5 for additional guidance on point combination and selection.

Lastly, it is important to address significant patterns of disharmony with the patient prior to more aggressive treatments with the eight extraordinary vessels. When a patient seeks acupuncture for fertility support, it is best to determine if the issue is more in the twelve primary meridians or whether one needs to employ the deeper vessels. Often, once a pattern of pathology is addressed, the patient can become pregnant. For example, severe Liver qi stagnation might be the issue, and once addressed, the patient can become pregnant. It is important to remember that for a variety of reasons some women are more fertile than others and there are other medical concerns to take into consideration before leaping into eight extraordinary vessel treatments. If the patient has been in acupuncture treatment and decides to pursue pregnancy, and it proves to be more difficult than originally considered, an eight extraordinary vessel treatment can be readily employed. However, if the patient has never had acupuncture and seeks fertility treatment (obviously because she is having a difficult time getting pregnant), it is prudent to treat any patterns the practitioner determines prior to employing the eight extraordinary vessel strategies.

It is not necessary to pair Ren Mai and Chong Mai for female fertility. Should the practitioner decide to take a more conservative approach, starting on either vessel can be helpful and productive. For example, treating the Ren Mai with low CV points and moxa might be the best approach. Again, once the patient is pregnant, the practitioner would not continue treating the eight extraordinary vessel(s). Chinese herbs can also be helpful for conception purposes.

When treating for sustaining pregnancies—that is, the patient can easily become pregnant but has a history of miscarriages—the treatment strategy and approach is similar. In this case, it is more important to address any patterns the practitioner discerns first before employing the eight extraordinary vessels. For example, if the patient has heat signs, this could be leading to the miscarriages, and the practitioner would want to address the heat condition first. Medications and chronic conditions need to be clearly understood. If the patient is on thyroid medication or medications for high blood pressure, for example, these conditions are a variable in the overall landscape of the patient. Also, if the patient has a genetic condition of a blood disorder or autoimmune condition, these too are factors to consider when addressing pregnancy sustainment. There are several blood disorders that conventional medicine has not yet been able to diagnose, and the patient's tongue—something acupuncturists pay more close attention to for diagnostic purposes—may not present the condition clearly. Blood stagnation and/or blood deficiency is often easy to determine based on tongue diagnosis. However, if a patient has a genetic coagulation disorder, for example, that is not necessarily a condition easily expressed on the tongue. In these cases, it is important to have a more integrative health approach with the patient, such as working with their obstetrician and midwife. Understanding laboratory results is more important in these particular fertility cases. In cases of problems with pregnancy sustainment, it can be beneficial to have the patient provide blood tests and laboratory results on a regular basis. With pregnancies that involve both male and female fertility concerns, often genetic testing can prove to be helpful.

As with other fertility strategies, once the patient becomes pregnant, the practitioner will want to stop the eight extraordinary vessel treatments and return to a treatment strategy following eight principle or five element theory, or perhaps a combination of both. While the eight extraordinary vessel treatments are a wonderful support in achieving conception and pregnancy, they can be dangerous once the patient is approaching their second to third week of pregnancy. As a general rule, at the moment of learning the patient is pregnant, stop the eight extraordinary vessel treatments; in some cases, the practitioner may want to advise the patient to cease using Chinese herbal formulas.

It has become more common to encounter patients who wish to undergo in vitro fertilization (IVF) or intrauterine insemination (IUI) treatments for pregnancy. As long as the patient is not yet pregnant, eight extraordinary vessel treatments can greatly enhance this process for pregnancy. Again, once the patient is pregnant, return to other theories of acupuncture for support and sustainment.

CHAPTER 12

THE ART OF PAIRING

Pairing in the context of the eight extraordinary vessel treatments has been a controversial topic. Li Shi Zhen taught pairing by stating that the eight extraordinary vessels are "not controlled by the 12 main channels nor are they arranged in exterior-interior combinations" (Chase and Shima, 2010, p.28). In other words, the fact that the Chong Mai and Yin Wei Mai share the same point combination does not automatically mean they should be paired.

Pairing has more to do with how the vessels work interdependently. The Yin and Yang Qiao Mai work so closely together that they are often paired based on how they function in the body and complement one another. The same is true for the Yin and Yang Wei Mai. Again, because they function in reciprocity within the body, there is a basis for their pairing. Pairing of the four primaries is a more advanced technique of the eight, and ideally not done hastily or without serious consideration.

Appropriate pairings of the primaries are as follows:

- Ren Mai and Du Mai. This is the most acceptable pairing of the primaries because of the Microcosmic Orbit and its relationship to internal cultivation. For more information, refer to Chapter 13.

- Chong Mai and Dai Mai. While this pairing is seemingly thrown together by default, they do complement one another. The Dai Mai is often referred to as the Belt or Girdle Vessel because of its horizontal trajectory around the body, binding all vessels together. It functions from the outside in, meaning that when the belt is too tight or too loose, the entire system is affected. By contrast, the Chong Mai can be viewed as an interior boundary because all the vessels have a relationship with the Chong Mai either directly or indirectly. Therefore, the Chong Mai can be seen as functioning from the inside out, while the Dai Mai functions from the outside in, thus creating a complementary relationship.

It is true that the eight extraordinary vessels contain excess from the twelve primary channels; however, the eight extraordinary vessels can exist with certain types of deficiencies; there can be mixed conditions. The vessels regulate blood and qi in the body and can be viewed as "overseers" of the body.

CHAPTER 13

THE MICROCOSMIC ORBIT

It has become commonplace to use the terms Ren Mai and Du Mai interchangeably when referring to the Conception Vessel (CV) and Governor Vessel (GV). However, this can mislead the new practitioner to believe that Ren Mai is the same as CV and Du Mai is the same as GV, when this is not actually the case. In classical texts, referring to the Ren Mai truly meant the Ren Mai, a channel system quite different from the CV. Likewise, Du Mai was true to its name, leaving modern practitioners to wonder about this discrepancy.

The eight extraordinary vessels can and should be used for physical-level symptoms. It is not incorrect or inappropriate to use them in this way; however, these vessels also have the potential to influence important facets of a person's life—the journey of the spirit. Li Shi Zhen was a strong believer in the concept of internal alchemy, which is a process by which one's spirit body becomes aware of karmic lessons and is able to transform its perceptions and relationship to the self and the world. In primeval times, it was depicted in pictures, not words. As modern-day physicians (acupuncturists and herbalists) evolved and discovered more about the extraordinary vessels, language was cultivated to describe these primal vessels which make up our true nature, thus resulting in the term "internal alchemy."

What is internal alchemy? Essentially, it is the process of achieving higher levels or states of being, in a spiritual context, not materialism— similar to what the Buddha described as "simply awake." The process of achieving or embarking upon internal alchemy practices causes one to let go of the more mundane and ordinary perspectives and to achieve a way of being that is lighter and more compassionate. This process leads to loving fully and unconditionally, and understanding the differences between conventional reality and ultimate reality. Regardless of achievement, simply attempting to cultivate internal alchemy will offer an internal peace of both mind and body, much like meditation, but to a greater extent. Meditation is only part of the process; austere yoga and mind training are also a part of the equation in terms of reaching the individual's highest potential as it relates to the spirit. Yoga and other practices will help even skeptical individuals. Understanding internal alchemy outside of new-age ideas is important for the practitioner to grasp when working with patients who seek higher levels of being.

Meditation practices, austere yoga, and other practices can be enhanced and complemented by activating the Microcosmic Orbit, which is the energetic orbit of the Ren Mai and Du Mai. They connect end-to-end in the body at the perineum and in the face, which are critical and vulnerable areas of the body as they are transition points within the functioning of the orbit (see Figure 13.1).

The Microcosmic Orbit is activated whether the Ren Mai and Du Mai are paired or addressed individually in treatment. If the intention of the practitioner is to fully cultivate and activate the circuit in the patient, then pairing them would be recommended; however, if the intention is more for physical-level symptoms or pathology relating to either the Ren Mai (bonding) or Du Mai (collapse of yang), then activating them consecutively and individually is recommended.

Pairing the Ren Mai and Du Mai—both primary vessels of the eight extraordinary vessels—should not be done on someone who is not emotionally stable and well supported by friends and family. If the practitioner believes the pathology lies within the vessels that comprise the Microcosmic Orbit, then it is best to treat the vessels individually according to the protocol outlined in Chapter 4, and after completing them individually, begin the pairing sessions. This provides for a more compassionate and thoughtful treatment process.

Li described the potential of internal alchemy as states of stillness, emptiness, and nonbeing. This level of awareness can seem far-fetched to the more literal-minded individual. However, for those who embark upon the spiritual journey of becoming more awake to the discernment of realities, learning how to have more states of stillness can be quite liberating.

The process of arriving at a state of nonbeing is referred to as the internal alchemy path. A combination of therapies to rid the body of pathology, spiritual deficiencies, and obstructions of the mind opens the path to higher states of awareness. To reiterate, it is a process and one that can take years to cultivate. The work accomplished through acupuncture treatments on the eight extraordinary vessels, followed by the intentional pairing of the Ren Mai and Du Mai with the purpose of activating and clearing the Microcosmic Orbit, is helpful to the individual seeking this level of change and evolution.

Stillness is a concept that may be somewhat easier to grasp, and more commonly discussed in modern society than the concepts of emptiness and nonbeing, which in themselves are not concepts. They are neither existent nor non-existent, but these conversations are difficult to hear and bear without proper training. Even if one were to practice stillness, that alone would bring enormous benefit and health to the individual. In modern-day society, it is commonplace to rush, living a life matched against an agenda or list, in constant reaction to past or future events. Being in the present moment can be more difficult. However, over time and with practice the individual can cultivate this stillness, and acupuncture can assist immeasurably, especially once the patient and practitioner have embarked upon the eight extraordinary vessel protocols.

Adhering to meditative practices leads one to the experience of stillness. It could be that the individual is so ridden with anxiety they need to start with a more active meditation, such as a walking meditation, swimming meditation, or a more contemplative meditation prior to sitting on a cushion, gazing gently forward, and focusing on the breath. When one can achieve this level of meditation, the breath begins to stabilize the mind. It is a fundamental process in taming the mind. When the individual is focusing solely upon the breath, the Orbit becomes engaged, and slowly the mind is tamed; thoughts begin to fall away. In the beginning, mental activity slows down, but over time it will eventually become so slow that thoughts never arise as distractions to the meditator. This process can take years to cultivate, but starting somewhere and practicing daily offers the best opportunity to achieve results.

It can be helpful for the seeker to practice meditation on the treatment table while the Ren Mai and Du Mai are activated through acupuncture. Guided meditations can be useful in relaxing the individual; however, they do not fully engage the Microcosmic Orbit or lead to higher levels of internal alchemy per se, because the verbal nature of guided meditations may tempt the ordinary mind to wander and follow conceptions. Therefore, they are more beneficial and helpful in stabilizing the mind as an individual's introduction to meditation. Further mind training, yoga, and focused breathing, including proper posture, are important to stimulate the yang energy to circumambulate with the yin energy, thereby activating the Microcosmic Orbit.

Before further explanation regarding the idea of emptiness and internal alchemy, it is important to understand a few specifics regarding the orbit. How does it actually work in the body?

There are approximately 35 different kinds of fluids found in the human body. Conventional medicine organizes these fluids into groups and categories based on function and location. For the purposes of understanding the flow of "essential air and fluids" as it relates to the eight extraordinary vessels, more specifically the Microcosmic Orbit, this chapter discusses primarily the breath (i.e., the essential air) and the essential fluids, including blood, cerebrospinal fluids, and pelvic secretions (semen and vaginal fluids). Splitting hairs would be mentioning serum and plasma in terms of blood; however, there is no need to go into minute detail regarding the breakdown of the fluids. Primarily, it is important to understand what fluids are involved regarding the Orbit when activated. More important to understand is the movement of essential air, or breath because it is the breath that is the powerhouse—the gears that move the flow of both jing and qi in the Orbit.

Before discussing air/breath and body fluids, it is prudent to mention the value and benefit of water. It is critical the individual is not dehydrated during the course of treating the eight extraordinary vessels, but most especially if treating the vessels that can activate the Orbit. The simple reason is that human beings are mostly water, ranging from about 75 percent in children and 50–60 percent in adults. The distribution of water throughout the body varies from organ to organ and tissue to tissue, with the brain and kidneys possessing the highest proportions of water. This is especially important as it relates to the Orbit because it is the flow of jing (coming from the Kidneys) and qi within the spinal fluid traveling through the brain that activates the mind's ability to function within the Orbit, to achieve the higher state of awareness. As the essential air and fluids descend along the Ren Mai, the essence of air and fluids travel through the Heart and return to the pelvic cavity before rising again through the Kidneys (see Figure 13.1).

Should the individual not have enough water in the body, these organs struggle to function physically and spiritually, thus potentially blocking the ability to activate or benefit from the Orbit in activation. This also explains why water is essential in all kinds of meditations; the kidneys and the brain need water. As a note, the heart and lungs have the next highest proportion of water.

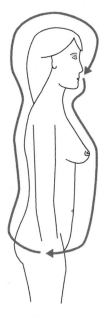

Figure 13.1 The Microcosmic Orbit

Although treating the eight extraordinary vessels can benefit the physical body, the true strength of the vessels is in promotion of the spiritual axis located deep in the body. The physical, emotional/mental, and spiritual body all rest within the confines of the physical body; however, it is the spirit and essence of the individual that gives rise to the physical and emotional conditioning. Given this rule of theory, treating the eight extraordinary vessels also treats the physical body. The anecdote of someone dying from a broken heart most resembles the explanation; the physical heart is fine, but the spirit of the heart is so broken, the body begins to fail.

As an interesting note, several Eastern exercises and activities involve the activation of the Microcosmic Orbit because of its ability to enable alchemy—a balance of the elements in an individual. Those familiar with Taoist traditions or activities, including forms of exercise, know intimately the functions of the Orbit. It is not new material to them.

In fact, there is documentation that discusses the functions and health of the Microcosmic Orbit dating to as early as the fourth century. There is no consensus on the exact time in history the I Ching in its original texts was first communicated; however, the Buddha (5th century) discussed many breathing techniques employing the Orbit while achieving a state of enlightenment. The I Ching is the oldest divination system in the world and is often used in the context of acupuncture—the hexagram system.

Jing and qi are often described as moving upward on the yin side and downward on the yang side. However, in the eight extraordinary vessels, jing and qi can flow in both directions. The flow of energy within the orbit travels upward on the yang side and downward on the yin side. This flow enables jing and qi to travel up through the spinal column and back side, coming from the depths of Kidney essence, through the brain for space and expansion of the mind, and descending through the Ren Mai, nourishing all of yin; the cycle continues while the individual is in the practice of orbit activation.

During the course of an eight extraordinary treatment, especially when Ren Mai and Du Mai are paired (deep and advanced treatment), the orbit is activated while the patient is on the treatment table. However, this activation can continue (with needles removed) for up to several days. If the individual can capitalize upon this activation by daily meditation, it is possible for advanced spiritual accomplishment, awakening, or a small step in evolution of the higher consciousness. There are also practices the individual can do at home or a place of their choosing that activate the orbit; yoga postures help enhance the activation. Many Taoist practitioners regularly participate in these types of yoga. Acupuncture and treating on the eight extraordinary vessels is only one method of orbit activation.

Lastly, even if the individual is not necessarily interested in activating the orbit for some type of spiritual advancement, activation of the orbit also enhances vital energy. Vital energy is used to produce true vitality. Vitality is something that benefits everyone regardless of the spiritual aspect. Once the orbit is in motion and the essential air and fluids are circulating optimally, the energies begin to replenish the body, harmonizing and reforming what is necessary for optimal health. The energy begins to produce vital fluids in the physical body, and combined with normal everyday energy, vital energy becomes more of the norm for the individual, which creates lifelong vitality. Naturally, this is a practice the individual needs to sustain regularly.

Emptiness is a more difficult concept for the ordinary person to comprehend. Emptiness is essentially a state of being, with an in-depth understanding of the differences between conventional reality (what our senses tell us) and ultimate reality, which is the navigation of our lives based on the consequences of our karma and karmic connections. Because free will exists, we have the ability to change and influence our karmic consequences for this life and future lifetimes. The individual can learn more about this idea of emptiness and how it is cultivated from the teachings of the Buddha and Tibetan Buddhist philosophy. For the purposes of this book, as it relates to the Microcosmic Orbit, it is best to understand that the Orbit has the capacity to allow the individual to achieve high states of awareness, through the combination of meditative practices, austere yoga, a healthy lifestyle, and acupuncture.

Li studied extensively with yoga masters, Buddhists, Daoists, and other more spiritually awakened teachers to understand the Orbit thoroughly. This is a good way to go about understanding emptiness and nonbeing. For now, while on the Earth and evolving, we can focus on being still, sitting, contemplating, and being *in* the world but not *of* the world.

The Microcosmic Orbit, fully activated, engages all three jiaos of the body: the upper with breath, the middle with process and dispersion of breath, and the lower with receiving and participating with breath. In the context of the Orbit, the breath moves up the Du Mai and down the Ren Mai, circulating in this manner. Through the process of being treated with the Orbit protocol, the individual returns to stillness, the original state of being, and is able to express externally the reclaiming of one's destiny in their life.

Li talked extensively about the importance of the practitioner (the physician) doing this work individually, prior to supporting the patient. He strongly believed that in order for the practitioner to truly help their patients, they must do the work first. This does not necessarily mean the practitioner must wait before giving treatments, but it does mean it is an ongoing process for both practitioner and patient. A key ingredient in this process is the practitioner's listening skills. In order to perceive things clearly, the listener must be able to be attentive without preconceived or discursive thoughts. This can take time to cultivate, but through meditative practices, practitioner treatments, and mind training, the practitioner is able to reach their highest potential and support patients in reaching theirs as well.

From a Tibetan Buddhist philosophical perspective, and in Li's descriptions, emptiness in the context of treatments is misunderstood most of the time. Emptiness does not mean nothing exists, nor is it synonymous with nothingness. It means phenomena do not exist in the way the conditioned mind thinks they do or should. The Dalai Lama explains emptiness as "the true nature of things and events," further urging the reader to "avoid the misapprehension that emptiness is an absolute reality or an independent truth" (Gyatso, 2015, pp.114–115).

Emptiness is not Heaven, nor a God-like realm separate from our world. All phenomena come from the five elements, and phenomena in their own existence are empty in their nature. Everything we experience is interdependent with something else; therefore, no phenomenon stands on its own. Everything is a temporary expression of one seamless and changing landscape. So, while emptiness can have a negative connotation in ordinary terms, within the context of internal alchemy, obtaining emptiness is liberation from suffering.

> For this reason, those who practice medicine and know of the Eight Vessels comprehend the great purpose of the 12 channels and 15 networks. Those who practice transcendence and know of the Eight Vessels miraculously attain the ascent and descent of the tiger and dragon, and the subtle aperture of the Mysterious Female. (Li Shi Zhen, cited in Chase and Shima, 2010, p.65)

In this context, Li is referring to the dragon as yang qi and the tiger as yin qi. He stated that the goal of internal alchemical cultivation is to promote the optimal interpenetration of yin and yang, meaning that yin is yang, and yang is yin. Ultimately, there is no separation. Lao Zi (Laozi, Lao Tzu), an ancient Chinese philosopher and writer, founder of philosophical Taoism, further described the dragon as the intellect and the tiger as desire, meaning that internal alchemical cultivation is the act of subduing the dragon and taming the tiger. "The valley spirit never dies; this is called the Mysterious Female" (Laozi, cited in Chase and Shima, 2010, p.187). The Mysterious Female is described by both Laozi and Li Shi Zhen as "the evocation of emptiness that gives birth to all things, and it is an allusion to the development of breath control as the vehicle for achieving the regulation of the ascent and descent of the dragon and tiger" (Chase and Shima, 2010, p.65).

In other words, one who knows of the eight extraordinary vessels and practices medicine can help patients obtain the knowledge regarding the functioning and spirit of the channels and networks within the body. However, those who are practicing medicine, know of the extraordinary vessels, *and are able to subdue the mind and tame desire*, not only achieve internal alchemy for themselves but can help their patients achieve internal alchemy. This control over the dragon and tiger comes about by being able to control the ascent and descent of breath through the Microcosmic Orbit by subduing the mind and taming desire. At the place of activation lies the Mysterious Female; in other words, the vital point (aperture) of this ascent and descent is the Mysterious Female. With sufficient time and dedicated practice, one can achieve transcendence.

Internal alchemy exists on a continuum. The detailed explanation of the Microcosmic Orbit and Mysterious Female is aligned with spiritual cultivation and higher degrees of awareness.

In order to achieve internal alchemy, we have to experience the world and witness our minds interact with the world, so that we can gather insight regarding what needs fixing. If we do not see ourselves in relation with other beings, how do we know what our emotional capacities might be? Living in a vacuum does not show us anything about ourselves. When we live in a cave, we could fancy ourselves to be great and enlightened beings. We could delude ourselves as to how kind and loving we are and be unable to understand why anyone might challenge us or disagree with our thoughts, decisions, and so on.

It is in our best interest to engage with the world: to be *in* the world, but not *of* the world. When in relationship with others, it is possible to observe our minds and emotions and to investigate them fully. Internal alchemy requires our willingness to see our faults, weaknesses, and states of confusion. And participation in the world lends us the opportunity to change, improve, and evolve in response to these observations. Internal alchemy cannot exist without the experiences of the world.

CHAPTER 14

HAVING FAITH

I t is important to remember that everyone heals uniquely and on their own timeline. Practitioners can be eager to see results and rush for measurements of success. The measurements of success are there, but often subtle. Healing occurs on a continuum. Some patients will have profound movements right away, while others will take a year, maybe longer, before showing signs of improvement regarding changes in emotion or on a spiritual plane. Physical changes will be more noticeable and generally occur sooner. Facilitating shifts in perception does not work quickly; it takes time and patience.

In fact, the biggest changes occur over time, little by little. A simple change in schedule or decision to wear a different color never worn before can be signs of subtle movement in qi or perspective, or both. It is important not to judge or become critical regarding an individual's progress as they move across the continuum of healing and change.

Have faith in the vessels, even if you struggle with having faith in your skill, competence, or education. If you are spot on with your point location, the vessels will activate, and you can have faith in the medicine. Acupuncture in general has one mission and that is to move a person toward health and wellbeing. Activating the eight extraordinary vessels invites a person to evolve beyond health and wellbeing: they offer the unique opportunity for the person to release the ties that bind them in their life, as well as future lives. Activating them releases obstacles of past lives to clear the way for growth and development. This sounds lovely. Who could possibly say no to being treated on these vessels? The truth is that growth and self-awareness come over time with a lot of effort and diligence, navigating the course no matter what. Often that means allowing emotional pain to rise, acknowledging the pain, and cultivating the highest level of self-integrity and development in the name of a more peaceful, balanced life with contentment.

Originally, practitioners treated these vessels over time, working with a strategy, iteration after iteration, returning to each vessel again and again. Then starting all over again.

CHAPTER 15

DIFFERENT STYLES

I n all fairness, there are several approaches to employing the eight extraordinary vessels. There is no right or wrong way, only different approaches depending on the intention of the practitioner, the constitution of the patient, and the goals for the treatment strategy.

This book primarily prescribes a more classical tradition of the philosophy and treatment planning. It certainly does not assert to be the only method of employing this theory in practice. Some theories suggest that only the master point is needed, and the couple point is merely an option. Especially as a novice practitioner, in determining whether to use the MP alone, or to add its CP, consider the following: while intention is certainly powerful, as beginners in a vast medicine it may prove difficult to know what is happening within the patient based on the intuition of the practitioner and their intention alone. Therefore, it may be best to subscribe to a proven method for both the healing of the patient, and the learning of the practitioner. Using only the MP of the vessel could be perceived simply as treating a single point unilaterally. Treating both the MP and its CP, the practitioner can be confident they have activated the extraordinary vessel.

It is up to the discretion of the practitioner to decide whether to use only those trajectory points which lie on the extraordinary vessel, or to target "off-trajectory points." With experience comes discernment.

Let us define trajectory points. As previously discussed, the MP and its CP activate the vessel. Along this pathway (also known as a trajectory) there are several other specific points the practitioner can access to facilitate the intention of the treatment. These points are selected based on patient complaints, pulse and tongue readings, and clinical observations both objective and subjective. In addition to specific points found on the pathway of each eight extraordinary vessel, there are other points not necessarily found on the pathway that can be useful during the treatment. These points are defined as "off-trajectory points."

How does a practitioner decide between trajectory points and off-trajectory points? The trajectory points both on the vessel trajectory as well as off the trajectory have a more profound effect and impact on the patient due to their relationship with the respective extraordinary vessel. This book contains a few off-trajectory points and their meaning/effect on the patient based on the extraordinary vessel. However, this list is not exhaustive and is offered as a starting point based on clinical experience.

It is also possible to focus on a meridian in the context of an extraordinary vessel. For example, there may be a case in which the practitioner is interested in treating points on the Gallbladder meridian for the purpose of addressing hip pain, the patient's inability to move forward in life and make decisions along the way, and an excessively teary and emotional disposition. The practitioner could consider the possibility of opening the Yang Qiao Mai for its effects on the physical structure of the person's body and its ability to incite optimism. Selecting points both on and off the Yang Qiao Mai trajectory, such as GB30, with Ashi points GB34, GB40, and GB1, would begin to alleviate the patient's complaints. This combination of points would address the physical complaints, while allowing the patient to form new perceptions and an optimistic outlook and move forward with decision making to support the long-range vision. If there is excessive heat in the meridian or pervasive heat in the patient, SI3 with other Small Intestine points could also be useful in releasing heat and assisting in sorting decisions, should that be needed.

Learning point combinations within the context of the extraordinary vessels takes time, experience, training, and discipline. It is strongly encouraged that the practitioner receive treatments on the extraordinary vessels systematically, diligently, with purpose and consistency, prior to treating others. In order for the practitioner to grasp the esoteric nature and full potential of the eight extraordinary vessels, it may require them to experience several iterations of treatment on the extraordinary vessel. However, at least one iteration is encouraged prior to the practitioner employing this treatment strategy on others.

The olden philosophy encourages practitioners to treat patients with the extraordinary vessels consistently throughout the treatment plan—in other words, flow through them in a systematic way, repeating the process, each time going deeper and doing more advanced treatments. Traditionally, this style of treatment strategy was perceived as a companion to longevity and wellbeing, offering access to a higher quality of life and higher levels of self-awareness. The treatment strategy engenders growth and wisdom, while addressing present-day complaints and simultaneously releasing past-life traumas to promote optimism for the healthy progression of future lives.

There are multiple approaches to treating the eight extraordinary vessels, including the option to use the MP alone or to add its CP. In developing one's stance on the matter, it is essential to have a deeper understanding of the activation process.

First, there remains controversy among practitioners not only regarding the point system but with regard to the use of trajectory points, how many to use and for how long, and how many times to open/close a vessel before proceeding to the next. It requires the practitioner to accept there are multiple ways to approach the theory, and the most important component is for the practitioner to be grounded in the theory and method they choose to employ with their patients.

This book focuses on a systematic method of approaching the treatments to support the practitioner in developing confidence and gaining wisdom and respect while working with the eight extraordinary vessels for the benefit of the patient.

Li Shi Zhen did not always use the current textbook MP and CP, but he did use a two-point system. He believed it was important to use a master and couple point to fully activate the vessel. Other advanced practitioners and those deemed "masters of the theory" use a two-point system. The primary criticism of the one-point system—that is, MP only—is that the MP is not sufficient to fully activate the vessel. Using a one-point approach is not wrong, and there are a host of practitioners who subscribe to this method; however, many advanced practitioners who are well versed in the use of the extraordinary vessels advise a two-point system to fully engage these deeper pathways.

It is important to understand point selection and needle action as a method of communicating to the energetic body. The point system and needle action are an opportunity for the practitioner to send a message to the patient's energy field at the deepest level.

Li Shi Zhen's two-point system involved the use of points that today would be called trajectory points on the eight extraordinary vessels.

Therefore, the modern-day point system does not differ from Li Shi Zhen's in its efficacy. The established master and couple point system used today has proven its potency over centuries.

Further, simply inserting the needles with an "even technique" and allowing the energetic body to assimilate and heal using its own wisdom has been proven to work for centuries. No needle action is necessary.

Novice practitioners to this theory are encouraged to learn more advanced techniques of the eight extraordinary vessels; however, it is important to have a starting point for the purposes of learning, and for the benefit of the patient. Therefore, having an established protocol is helpful for both practitioner and patient. Again, this book is a starting point for practitioners to begin the process of integrating the extraordinary vessels into their treatment plans, with the understanding they will continue to grow and learn from these treatments for many years. There are, of course, several advanced techniques and styles to adopt along the way. This book is intended to provide a basic protocol for a novice to the theory. Ideally, a practitioner will learn from every extraordinary vessel treatment provided, continually deepening their understanding of the inner workings of the energetic system.

—— CHAPTER 16 ——

A LUCID ACCOUNT

The Qiao Mai are beautifully orchestrated and choreographed to meet the current life structure. These vessels govern what is left to right and right to left. They act as a capsule of sorts, containing the mind and conceptual thoughts; in health, they stave off overthinking and repetitive thought patterns, including habits. Out of balance, the Qiao Mai may foster obsession, irrational thought, and extremist viewpoints. They are instrumental in human structure, governing gait and outer expression of movement.

The Wei Mai are the "gushy" part inside of the individual. Think of the Qiao Mai and Wei Mai as a crab—hard on the outside, mushy on the inside. The Qiao Mai are the structure to hold the Wei Mai together. The Wei Mai are the tapestry of our lives, the emotions, past-life memories, our process with accepting what is happening in life. The Wei Mai hold past-life memories that impact the current life, obstructing evolution and blocking movement forward. The tapestry is correct yet fluid and adaptable, changing as life unfolds.

Think of the Qiao Mai and Wei Mai as a unit. Hugely misunderstood and underused, they can treat everything related to this life, including the present moment and past-life memories that are lodged deep in the consciousness. These vessels are in a constant state of assessment of the outer and inner worlds: what is safe, what is not safe, what can be trusted, what cannot be trusted. They are always referring back to a past memory for data collection and intelligence gathering.

The Chong Mai holds the individual's world view and is central to a way of thinking and behaving in the world. It is filled with imprinting of past- and current-life moldings, experiences, traumas, and memories locked in the body. It governs perceptions and adaptability, fertility, belief, and faith in what is just. It is sexual, compassionate, bliss-filled, and in touch with the consciousness's larger scheme of what is meant to unfold.

Everyone can benefit from better, more connected, and enriched interpersonal relationships. At the depths of our being we want to be loved unconditionally, and accepted for who we are, regardless of color, sex, faith, preferences, and way of life. How we bond with our parents and siblings is a result of the Ren Mai, and that gets carried into our interpersonal relationships as adults. This is where breakdown most likely occurs. What happens in the first few moments of our introduction to life, whether it be at home or in a hospital, farmland or table, in the cab or on the living-room couch, creates a path that can never be repeated. The energetic dynamic between mother and child is so crucial yet highly undervalued in modern times. Those first few years are a period of imprinting, introduction, and indoctrination into this life, at this time, in this realm. The domain of Ren Mai asks: Are we present, are we really there, are we accepted and loved, and how do we look? How do we feel about our family? Are we in a family?

The Ren Mai holds the key to the path of interpersonal relationships and the ability to evolve, progress, and proceed with life's plan. If one has a strong Du Mai to accompany the Ren, then most individuals succeed. In short, the Ren Mai is about bonding and relationships, including one's relationships with the self. It is about family, children, fertility, sex, intimacy, and connecting to something outside of the self-effacing ego.

Given that the Du Mai is about moving in the world, music, dance, flow, qi, possession, and confidence, it is important that the Du Mai supports the weaknesses of the Ren Mai. Together they can overcome many traumatic experiences, cultivate forgiveness, and move forward in a healthy manner. If both are damaged, the Orbit is damaged. This results in compromised mental health, manifesting across a continuum from subtle to advanced degrees of mental deficiencies.

The gutter, where everything goes when it is not resolved, describes the Dai Mai. It is the holder of all that is in excess and non-serving. Physically, it can manifest as weight, but not everyone who has pathology in the Dai Mai is overweight. The excess can be physical, emotional, or spiritual. It is the gutter of not only the physical body but of the mind. It is fear, worry, and the ties that bind. Sometimes the individual thinks and feels they have let go of a situation, person, or circumstance, but the memory can get lodged in the Dai Mai, held in the gutter, and create blockages to moving forward. Think of it as a gutter that needs cleaning out; in some cases, it may only be partially blocked, so there is a minimal degree of movement forward. The individual may describe feeling unable to fully move on or forward, and find it difficult to understand, believing they have dealt with the trauma or situation.

CHAPTER 17

CASE STUDIES

CASE STUDY 1

The patient is in her early 70s and maintains a good diet and exercise regime. She drinks plenty of water and measures it daily to ensure she receives adequate amounts. She is in good health, maintains a healthy weight, and possesses normal strength for her age and gender. Tongue presentation initially showed deficient heat signs. The tongue picture matched that of Qiao Mai pathology as described in Chapter 1, initially red in color. The pulse picture included a tightness on the Liver meridian with a tapping quality and choppy. This further confirmed Qiao Mai pathology.

The patient is married and has children and grandchildren whom she sees regularly. After a long and successful career in education, she is now retired. The patient maintains regular acupuncture treatments and has been in treatment for approximately two years.

The patient was given positive feedback from a co-worker who was receiving acupuncture treatments, and recommended the patient try it for her hip pain. In an effort to maintain good health and discover if acupuncture would help with her pain, she decided to make her first appointment. Primary complaints included joint stiffness specifically in her upper back and neck. The patient has a history of minor surgeries and the removal of a non-Hodgkin's lymphoma on the back of her scalp, just lateral to the semispinalis capitis in the region of the splenius capitis muscle group of the scalp on the right side. She underwent radiation treatment, and although she has had a clean health report since the procedure, approximately six months after the radiation treatments, she experienced a sharp pain in the area of the procedure that would come and go randomly. She reported she could not discern a pattern of behavior, food, or lifestyle event that would trigger the sharp pain which was becoming more chronic.

The patient received three treatments focused on the movement of qi and blood prior to employment of Yin Qiao Mai paired with Yang Qiao Mai. She was in good health, maintaining a good diet with plenty of exercise. After receiving these treatments, she reported significant improvement with sleep, increased range of motion in her hips, less joint stiffness overall, and her anxiety—mostly from long-term work-related stress—appeared to be manageable. However, she continued to experience chronic pain at the base of her scalp on the right side that would become sharper at random times of the day. The sharpness could last as long as one or two hours, but most often the sharpness lasted for several minutes before becoming dull.

Her first Qiao Mai treatment included the MP and CP of both Qiao Mai, trajectory points GB20 and GV15, off-trajectory point GB34, and versatile points SI3 and 8 (see Chapters 5 and 6 for further description of points).

The Qiao Mai treatment with similar point combinations was employed for a total of eight treatments. With each treatment, the patient reported significant improvement. Improvement included decreased sharp pains during the day, less chronic and dull pain, and more range of movement in her neck. In fact, there were some days where she felt no pain. When the pain returned, it seemed to be less intense and last only for a few seconds to a minute in duration.

Given that the patient had significant improvement, the next "phase" of eight extraordinary vessel treatment was pursued. After finishing one complete iteration of the eight extraordinary vessels, a return to the Qiao Mai, paired, began. The patient reported significant improvement in all areas of her life. The patient further reported she noticed a difference in how she feels emotionally and is more able to manage the stressors in her life. After completing one full iteration of the eight extraordinary vessels, the patient no longer experienced the pain in her scalp.

After the initial Qiao Mai treatments, and one complete iteration of the eight extraordinary vessels, the patient received an additional 20 treatments on the Qiao Mai, paired. This meant that after treating all eight extraordinary vessels according to the prescribed protocol, the patient received an additional 20 treatments on the Qiao Mai with varying trajectory, off-trajectory, and versatile point combinations based on tongue and pulse presentations, and the patient's report of symptoms.

Two years after the patient's first eight extraordinary vessel treatment, she reports almost no pain anywhere in her body except occasional stiffness resulting from a wrong movement or overuse of an arm or knee, for example. Further, she has only experienced one scalp pain episode and believes that was the result of dehydration.

Final comments

This patient initially received approximately three treatments to move qi and blood using a TCM method of treatment prior to her first eight extraordinary vessel treatment. She received eight Qiao Mai (paired) treatments. After completing the eight Qiao Mai treatments, one complete iteration of the eight extraordinary vessels was employed. After one complete iteration of the extraordinary vessels, a return to the Qiao Mai (paired) with off-trajectory and versatile point combinations was employed. The patient receives Qiao Mai treatments regularly to maintain an active and healthy lifestyle. The trajectory and versatile point combinations fluctuate treatment to treatment depending upon what the patient reports and tongue and pulse readings. The Qiao Mai functions include binding the left and right sides of the body, with a focus on maintaining the structure of muscles. This makes them uniquely qualified to assist with any aspect of the structure of the body. Additionally, they mostly work with the post-natal qi, meaning they influence present life and present-day activities. Lastly, they influence the Wei Mai and have a close relationship with the Ren Mai and Du Mai, yin and yang, respectively. As a result, this patient is able to maintain an integration of her medical history with current life events while creating a positive and active life. The health of the physical body creates space for the growth of the mind and spirit.

───── CASE STUDY 2 ─────

The patient is in her early 40s and maintains a good diet and exercise regime. While she attempts to drink adequate amounts of water, she currently drinks approximately 20 ounces of Diet Coke daily, and wine most evenings with dinner. She is in good health, maintains a healthy weight, and possesses above-average strength for her age and gender. The patient's medical history includes a significant ankle surgery on the right side when she was younger and with a successful recovery. Her initial tongue presentation included a slightly white coat except in the Large Intestine area where it was more yellow. Her tongue was wide and thin, appearing redder in the area of Liver and Gallbladder. Her pulses were overall low and deficient. The eight extraordinary pulse picture was difficult to determine. Although her pulses were deficient, there was a tightness and tenseness about them that most resembled either Qiao Mai or Dai Mai pathology. She is an avid runner, married, and has two small children (ages nine and four). She has held a demanding job for approximately 21 years. The patient maintains regular acupuncture treatments and has been in treatment for approximately five years.

The patient was given positive feedback from a co-worker who was receiving acupuncture treatments, and recommended the patient try it for fertility. The patient had been trying to have her second child for a few years without success. While her initial strategy was for fertility, after the initial intake it was apparent she would benefit from stress reduction and a consult regarding nutrition and exercise. The patient was running an excessive number of miles per week to manage her anxiety and stress, and although she ate in a healthy manner, she was consuming gluten, dairy, and sugars. Additionally, at that time she was consuming over 40 ounces of Diet Coke daily.

He primary complaint was suspected infertility. She reported there had not been any concerns with her first pregnancy and she was perplexed as to why having her second child was not "as easy."

The patient received four treatments focused on the movement of qi and blood, and blood deficiency prior to employment of the Yin Wei Mai. With the first three Yin Wei Mai treatments, the MP and CP point were used and trajectory point SP15. After three successful Yin Wei Mai treatments, the patient was experiencing stress reduction and open to lifestyle coaching. There were two additional treatments primarily focusing on the Kidney, Spleen, and Heart meridians and their sister meridians, prior to employing the Chong Mai.

She was in good health, maintaining a relatively good diet with plenty of exercise. Nutritional consults encouraged a variety of meats, to include 4–8 ounces of red meat weekly, vitamins, and plenty of green leafy vegetables. The running was draining her qi faster than she could replenish it, and therefore a compromise was reached regarding the number of miles she was running weekly. She was encouraged to incorporate yoga and an active form of meditation to help with her anxiety. The patient was receptive to consults. Prior to employing the Chong Mai strictly for fertility purposes, she reported significant improvement with sleep and energy, and her anxiety was becoming more manageable. The patient's tongue began showing signs that the blood deficiency pattern was improving, and her pulse picture improved with each treatment.

Her first Chong Mai treatment included the MP and CP, trajectory point KI16, and versatile point HT7. (See Chapters 5 and 6 for further description of points.)

This combination and similar point combinations was employed for a total of nine treatments, with the patient receiving acupuncture weekly. With each treatment, the number of trajectory and off-trajectory points was increased, not exceeding a total of 12 points. With each treatment, the patient reported significant improvement with sleep, managing her stress, having normal menstrual cycles, and generally feeling more capable of managing her personal and professional life. At her thirteenth treatment, she reported being pregnant; she felt both excited and slightly worried. The eight extraordinary vessel treatments were stopped, and a combined TCM and five element theory/method was started. Her healthy son was born at 38 weeks.

This patient continued to stay in acupuncture treatments post-delivery, and various ailments, aches, pains, and stressors were addressed during her treatments using a combined theory method. Her tongue picture began to show signs of Liver heat. During a routine medical visit that consisted of lab work, a high enzyme count on her liver function tests was revealed. A Chinese herbal formula was prescribed to support Liver functioning by harmonizing Liver qi and expelling heat in the blood.

Over the course of three years, most of her complaints were on the physical level. Occasionally, there were discussions of an emotional or spiritual nature. Although the treatments were consistently addressing physical complaints, points chosen within a combined theory always included points possessing a strong spiritual component to them such as upper Kidney points, the outer Bladder line, points on the Heart meridian, and CV14 and 15, for example. Given the patient is a Wood constitution in five element theory, most treatments were grounded and ended with command points on the Liver and Gallbladder meridians.

The patient accomplished a significant amount of emotional work during this time; however, four years after her first acupuncture treatment, she revealed deep emotional concerns regarding her personal life that were affecting her professional life. Not sure how to approach her situation, she engaged in an inappropriate relationship with a co-worker. Given that the patient had received over 100 treatments, and was doing well physically, the eight extraordinary vessel theory was employed once again to help support her emotional struggle while she worked on her relationship with her husband and feelings of self-worth and self-respect.

The patient received five Yin Wei Mai treatments that coincided with therapy treatments she received in couples counseling. The patient was also taking Chinese herbs to help with Liver functioning and her menstrual cycles. The herbs had a profound effect on stabilizing her mood, especially during her cycles. With the Yin Wei Mai treatments, the MP and CP were used, trajectory points SP15 and LR14, off-trajectory points KI16 and 19, and versatile points HT7 and GB39.

The intention with the Yin Wei Mai treatments was to support all yin meridians, help the patient develop trust (trust of self and trust of others), heal from being torn emotionally, and manage overwhelming daily anxiety. Balanced yin meridians help an individual keep life balanced day to day. The Yin Wei Mai has a unique way of impacting all yin meridians. At treatment number 127, the patient revealed she wanted to take a break from acupuncture to work with a shaman. She did not want to combine her sessions with a shaman with her acupuncture treatments, in order to obtain a true measurement of success, or not. After four months of visiting a shaman, the patient returned to acupuncture, reporting a good experience and an interest in learning how to be more appropriately "open" with people in general. The Wei Mai treatments were resumed.

Final comments

This patient received eight extraordinary vessel treatments early in treatment for a specific reason. Afterwards, she accumulated years of acupuncture treatments using a combined treatment method (TCM and five element acupuncture) before receiving eight extraordinary vessel treatments in a more traditional sense. The Yin Wei Mai treatments assisted the patient in developing more appropriate relationships in her personal and professional life. This patient was reportedly doing well up until a global crisis hit the world and her job became increasingly more stressful. In an effort to support her body, which is now older, the Qiao Mai are currently being treated. The intention will be to incorporate these treatments often and with consistency to help her navigate and manage post-natal qi and current work-related stressors causing excess tension. At some point, the Dai Mai will need to be treated, depending on the level of excess emotional stress.

CASE STUDY 3

The patient is in his early 40s. Diet, nutrition, and exercise were not something he initially paid enough attention to. However, after starting acupuncture he became receptive to dietary suggestions, increased his water intake, and began to exercise more regularly. He is in good health overall and maintains a healthy weight. Tongue presentation indicated blood deficiency in general, being pale to pink in color, slightly dry with a thin white coat, and with a small crack down the middle that is often referred to as a "stomach crack." Initially, his pulses were somewhat erratic and most resembled Chong Mai pathology. After the first two treatments, his pulses became more stable and would "fill" after each treatment.

The patient is married and has one child. He maintains regular acupuncture treatments and has been in treatment for approximately one and half years.

Initially, the patient's wife was in treatment for fertility reasons. The couple had not been successful in getting pregnant with their second child, and acupuncture was recommended as an alternative to try prior to IVF treatments.

Primary complaints included fertility support and help in managing stress levels. The patient reported no major surgeries or injuries; however, he had been diagnosed with varicocele. At the time he started acupuncture, he had not sought any type of conventional treatment for his condition.

The patient received five treatments focused on the movement of qi and blood with points primarily on the Liver and Spleen channels. In the five element tradition and theory, the patient is a Water constitution, and therefore many of the initial acupuncture treatments ended with tonifying command Kidney meridian points. After five treatments using a combined theory method (TCM and five element), the Yin Wei Mai paired with Yang Wei Mai was successfully employed for two treatments with trajectory points SP13 and 15, off-trajectory points LR9 and SP10, and versatile point KI9. After the Wei Mai treatments, the Chong Mai was employed. Typically, the practitioner would not rush with treating a "primary" extraordinary vessel; however, given that the patient was emotionally stable, reported no structural complaints or pain other than an occasional ache in his scrotum, and was content with his work and home life, there was no apparent obstacle to treating the Chong Mai after two successful treatments of the Wei Mai.

The Yin Wei Mai is also considered the "transition vessel" to the primary eight extraordinary vessels. In this case, the Chong Mai was employed intentionally for the purpose of fertility support.

At the time of starting the extraordinary treatments, the patient was in better health than at the first initial acupuncture treatment, and was regularly engaged in a healthy diet, exercise, and drinking adequate amounts of water. He reported feeling better overall, sleep had improved, and he felt less stressed in his day-to-day activities. Further, the occasional ache in his scrotum seemed to be improving.

His first Chong Mai treatment included the MP and CP, trajectory points KI13 and 15, off-trajectory points SP6 and CV5, and versatile point CV9. (See Chapters 5 and 6 for further description of points.)

This combination and similar point combinations were employed for a total of ten treatments, but not in sequence—after five treatments of the Chong Mai, the patient was treated for flu-like symptoms and the Chong Mai was not employed. Chong Mai treatments resumed after approximately two non-eight extraordinary vessel treatments for an additional five treatments.

Even though the patient was feeling generally well, and his wife was improving with her treatments, the couple still had not been able to get pregnant. Therefore, an updated semen analysis and evaluation of the varicocele condition was recommended. At treatment number 16, the Chong Mai was paired with the Ren Mai for approximately four treatments. At treatment number 21, the patient reported improvement with semen analysis findings, and while the varicocele showed signs of improvement, surgery was recommended. At this time, he started taking Chinese herbs, specifically a formula that focused on Kidney qi and Kidney yang.

The patient received an additional nine treatments on the Chong Mai after his surgery and continued his Chinese herbal formula. He recovered well and resumed normal activities within four weeks of his surgery. To assist with his healing while staying on track with the overall strategy, the fourth trajectory of the Chong Mai was employed, using the MP and CP, trajectory points Kidney 10 and 11, off-trajectory points SP3 and LR3, and versatile point SP6.

Final comments

One year after the patient started acupuncture treatments, his wife became pregnant. At the time of the pregnancy, his semen analysis showed significant signs of improvement and he experienced no scrotum pain or pain from his surgery. The patient continues to maintain healthy eating habits, is diligent with regular exercise, consumes adequate amounts of water, and continues taking his Chinese herbs. After a four-month break from acupuncture once his wife became pregnant, he resumed acupuncture treatments to maintain good health and support his immune system.

Hindsight is an important factor in the growth of the practitioner. This case study is a reflection of learning that a Chinese herbal formula might have proved productive had it been scripted earlier in the treatment strategy. The outcome was reached, but after a considerable amount of time.

CASE STUDY 4

The patient is in her late 40s. Diet, nutrition, and exercise continues to be a topic of conversation. The patient has tried many different types of diets, and while she understands the value of exercise, she does not follow a regular, consistent regime. Acupuncture treatments have included coaching with nutritional and dietary recommendations. The patient initially started acupuncture as part of her overall wellness plan. She struggles with maintaining a healthy weight and has consistently been in therapy to address emotional swings. She has a history of trauma and had a difficult relationship with her mother (who has since passed). Initially, her tongue presentation was wide and thick in size, dry, pale except at the Heart tip, which was red. In general, her pulses were deficient; most resembled Dai Mai pathology.

The patient is divorced from her one marriage and has no children. She maintains regular acupuncture treatments and has been in treatment for approximately seven years. She is a writer and a highly creative person, who enjoys cats and long walks. Her mind is generally open and expansive, and she describes herself as a spiritual person.

The general theme with this patient is centered around relationships—professionally, personally, and with herself. At her initial treatment, she reported multiple failed relationships and a difficult time staying employed.

The death of her father left her with a small inheritance, and she made the decision to embark upon a spiritual path to discover the themes in her life and how to best address the pathologies.

The seven years of acupuncture treatments disclose a long history of this patient having difficulty with interpersonal relationships that consistently interfere with her professional work and romantic relationships.

The patient initially received six treatments focused on the movement of qi and blood and resolving dampness which was pervasive. She suffered from sinus issues, irregular bowel movements, and fibroids. With the earlier treatments, she was emotional and teary, with the occasional rise of anger in her voice. After six treatments using a TCM theory method, the Yin Wei Mai was employed. At the time of starting the Yin Wei Mai treatments, the patient's tongue presented an improvement with the damp condition—not as swollen or pale. Further, she reported having more regular bowel movements.

It was at this time that the patient was diagnosed by conventional medicine as having a fibroid; the size required surgery for removal. She decided to undergo a partial hysterectomy, having only her uterus removed. Eight extraordinary vessel treatments stopped and a TCM method of treatment and scar treatments were used prior to resuming eight extraordinary vessel treatments, which were not employed again until her seventeenth treatment.

At acupuncture treatment number 13, the patient reported feeling emotional and "lost," and traveled to Nepal. Upon returning, she reported feeling more connected to her spiritual path and overall better about herself. At treatment number 17, the eight extraordinary vessel treatments resumed, starting with the Yin Wei Mai using the MP, CP, trajectory points KI9 and SP15, off-trajectory points SP8 and LR9, and versatile points HT7 and SP6 for two treatments before treating the Ren Mai at treatment number 20. A full and complete iteration of the eight extraordinary vessels was employed with short breaks between the Ren Mai, Du Mai, and Dai Mai.

The patient averaged four treatments per eight extraordinary vessel, and with each shift to the next vessel, the patient experienced tremendous but often painful emotional progress. Her body withstood minor aches, pains, and occasional bouts of irregular bowel movements. Although she changed therapists a total of three times over the course of seven years, she consistently sought therapy and spiritual retreats to help her manage the extreme emotional pain she was determined to address.

Final comments

This patient has achieved significant milestones over the course of treatments, including a large release of anger at treatment number 25 that expressed itself in heavy crying, a long spiritual retreat at treatment number 38, a change in diet to an "elimination" diet and focus on gut health at treatment number 41, and an increase in self-acceptance at treatment number 47.

At treatment 68, the patient started a Chinese herbal formula designed for stress and anxiety. Although the patient was improving, a common theme of difficulty in her relationships continued professionally and personally. However, at treatment number 78 she reported doing significantly better. She had incorporated the therapeutic model eye movement desensitization and reprocessing (EMDR) in her wellness regime to assist with managing her past trauma. She was finally addressing emotions that lived deeply in her body and were trapped in the tissue. Ready to release, she began to make significant improvement with her interpersonal relationships by treatment number 95.

With this case, the years of trauma were deeply buried in the fibers of her body. She received a total of 36 extraordinary vessel treatments over the course of several years. Her emotional growth has been substantial, and while she continues with acupuncture and therapy, her ability to maintain a job, have appropriate perspective, and engage in a romantic relationship has drastically improved. She can now discuss her traumas without anger, resentment, or complete breakdown; she can see them from an objective perspective and work with the emotions that surface as a result of her traumas.

CASE STUDY 5

The patient is a 49-year-old male who is in relatively good health, maintaining a healthy weight and conscientious about his health in general. Diet and nutrition are easily managed; however, exercise is difficult due to his diagnosis of psoriatic arthritis, osteoarthritis, and degenerative disc disease among many others in the area of arthritis. This patient was an athlete as a young person and young adult, and body composition remains strong. Most treatments have focused on physical ailments. Professionally, the patient is a psychologist and emotionally healthy and stable. He started acupuncture treatments and maintained regular visits for approximately two years. During this time, a variety of joint and tendon discomfort were treated primarily by using TCM methods.

After approximately two years of consistent treatments, the patient took a break from acupuncture. During this time, he visited a rheumatologist and started seeing a chiropractor regularly. After seven years, he returned to acupuncture. At the time of his return his tongue presentation was long, narrow, red, and dry. His pulses were full and pounding. Both his tongue and pulse presentation most resembled Qiao Mai pathology.

Prior to the seven-year hiatus, he had received 22 acupuncture treatments. In addition, during the time absent from acupuncture treatment he was receiving treatment in other modalities, including steroid injections primarily in his neck, shoulders, feet, and fingers. Given his emotional stability, upon his return to acupuncture treatments, the Qiao Mai (paired) were employed. These vessels have a direct influence on the body in terms of structure; therefore, the intention was to support the bones, muscles, and tendons as much as possible prior to directly influencing the arthritic conditions. After three successful treatments using the MP and CP, and various combinations of trajectory points SI10, LI15 and 16, BL59, and KI2, and versatile points GB39, TB5, and GV4, the Du Mai was employed. The patient was treated on the Du Mai multiple times using the MP and CP, and various combinations of trajectory points GV4, 8, 12, and 14. Off-trajectory points BL23–26, 39, and 40, and versatile points TB5, SI10, and SI11. The reasoning for treating the Du Mai was to assist in supporting adequate and appropriate spinal fluid movement servicing the nerves and nervous system.

This patient started receiving infusions and more steroid shots in order to manage his pain. The acupuncture treatments helped facilitate the effectiveness of the infusions and steroid shots. He continued to receive chiropractic care as well. The combination of this integrative approach enables him to live a seemingly normal life with only occasional discomfort. His strategy is important to maintain in order to "stay ahead" of the pain, rather than getting behind it and having to catch up.

The acupuncture also helps maintain immune support and mitigate side effects from the steroids. After his infusions and/or steroid shots, it can be difficult for him to sleep; he has more fluctuations in his weight (but not to the degree that it becomes problematic) and sweating, and, more recently, his blood pressure has been increasing. The acupuncture treatment strategy is to mitigate these side effects, in addition to immune support and pain management.

Final comments

This patient has received a total of 37 treatments since returning to acupuncture. Treatments have consisted of an ongoing approach of treating the Qiao Mai (paired) and the Du Mai, with TCM treatments in between treating the extraordinary vessels. This approach has supported successful clinical application of the theory. Without the integrative approach to his health care needs, the patient would be in chronic and at times debilitating pain. As a benefit of treating these vessels in tandem with other methods focused on pain management, the patient receives treatment that addresses hypertension, issues involving the endocrine system, and sleep disturbances. Additionally, treating these vessels supports his gait from a neurological standpoint, potentially mitigating diseases associated with "wind" conditions such as Parkinson's disease.

The treatments on the Du Mai support neurological functioning, perspective, and balancing states of overwhelm with a calmer disposition to life's ups and downs.

—————— CASE STUDY 6 ——————

The patient is a 68-year-old woman who initially came to acupuncture for support with weight loss. Clinically diagnosed with morbid obesity, she was concerned about her health and realized she needed help in addressing her weight challenges. Although her diet was relatively healthy, the issue resided in long-standing pathological emotional eating habits. She lives alone and is retired from a successful technological career, and currently enjoys painting, gardening, and writing poetry. She is a very talented artist and has developed a rewarding second career of selling her paintings and publishing a book of poetry. Initial tongue presentation indicated a pervasive damp condition; her tongue was wide, thick, slightly pale, and moist. Her pulses presented no blocks or abnormalities, and moderately full. Tongue and pulse presentation most resembled Dai Mai pathology.

The patient has been in regular acupuncture treatments for five years, receiving treatment approximately every two to three weeks consistently. In the first few treatments, it was determined that part of the weight gain was due to excruciating knee pain which made it difficult to walk or navigate stairs. The added weight contributed to the pain. She reported she often felt a disconnect between her head and the rest of her body, as if she was almost disengaged from her body below the neckline. Based on what the patient shared in the first few treatments, her emotional wellbeing was unhealthy, and she had repressed many traumatic memories, stemming from early childhood.

During the first year of treatment, TCM methods were employed for pain management, organ support (primarily her kidneys), and a lot of coaching with reframing thoughts and language. After a year of acupuncture, the patient was able to make an appointment regarding her knees, and over the course of the following two years she received double knee replacements—right knee and subsequently her left knee. She received acupuncture treatments prior to surgery as well as in her home post-surgery.

During the two-year period of managing knee surgery and the recovery process, the eight extraordinary vessels were employed systematically and consistently, starting with the Qiao Mai, one by one (i.e., not paired). After approximately three successful treatments of each Qiao Mai, the Wei Mai were employed in the same manner. A number of trajectory, off-trajectory, and versatile points were used in combination during these treatments. By the time the patient had recovered from the second knee replacement, all eight extraordinary vessels had been successfully employed in the following order: Qiao Mai, Wei Mai, Ren Mai, Du Mai (primary), Chong Mai (primary), and Dai Mai, both draining and consolidating depending on other symptoms. The off-trajectory points assisted with knee recovery while the intention of the extraordinary vessels was to support her emotional health to prevent further weight gain.

A tremendous amount of work regarding her emotional wellbeing took place during this time. She was able to reintegrate painful memories and eventually sought professional counseling. In addition, she was able to return to walking and navigating her stairs, and gardening. The ability to exercise helped her navigate the tricky waters of her eating habits. After a full iteration of the eight extraordinary vessels, the patient was able to openly discuss her overeating and the triggers associated with her binge habits. She reported finally being able to be in touch with her body beyond the neck down.

In her third year of treatment, the patient suffered from Meniere's disease and several reoccurring bladder and urinary tract infections that were diagnosed by lab work. She did not have noticeable pain or symptoms of the infections. This was concerning as most people experience discomfort or varying symptoms with these types of infections.

A second iteration of the eight extraordinary vessels was employed over the course of the next year in the same manner as the first iteration. With the second iteration of the extraordinary vessels, National Acupuncture Detoxification Association (NADA) protocols were included for food addiction, and an increased focus on the Liver meridian was added using off-trajectory points and versatile points in combination with the respective master and couple points. In the transitionary period from one extraordinary vessel to the next, a series of Lung and Heart points were used in order to bridge the functions of the Heart with its minister, the Lung meridian. The patient continued her cognitive therapy, and although she did not seem to lose considerable weight, her emotional work improved slowly over time. After a second full iteration of the extraordinary vessels, the patient reported having mended the bridge with her brother, her only living relative, and enjoying her new relationship with him. They were able to have communication that left her feeling joyful instead of angry and hurt. She was able to communicate with him her feelings about the past and how she wanted a different relationship with him.

As this patient progressed into her fourth year of acupuncture treatment, the infections seemed to improve and eventually stopped occurring. She still needs to move slowly when rising from lying down; however the Meniere's disease seems to have resolved itself. The patient reported being open to other modalities in order to help her integrate painful memories, get in touch with her body in a deeper, perhaps spiritual way, and continue the work with self-acceptance. While maintaining acupuncture treatments, the patient received a few treatments of hypnosis and attended group therapy sessions. After a series of these treatments, she decided to discontinue and return to cognitive therapy and acupuncture, and to see a nutritionist. Lab findings indicated she had fatty liver disease and an enlarged spleen. As a result, she started regular sessions with the nutritionist.

Final comments

This patient has made huge strides in her emotional health. Although she continues to struggle with her weight, her emotional/mental health improvement has been significant and is ongoing. Her ability to integrate her body, accept it, and appreciate what it has carried her through has been significant. She understands that the emotional work needs to take place before she can lose a significant amount of weight and keep it off in a healthy manner. She is aware of her triggers and can objectively watch herself make decisions based on her emotions—when she is eating for health and when she is eating to feed emotions.

She walks, gardens, and uses the stairs in her home for exercise. Leasing an art studio, she continues to paint and has built a community of artists around her. At some point, a third iteration of the extraordinary vessels will be of benefit. In the meantime, she is receiving Dai Mai treatments consistently with the NADA protocol and varying trajectory, off-trajectory, and versatile point combinations. She actively sees a therapist and nutritionist as well. Her weight loss has been minimal, but her knowledge of its presence and how it got there is profound.

CHAPTER 18

CONCLUDING REMARKS

Judgment of phenomena yet knowing phenomena are illusory begs the question "How do we navigate the movie of our lives?" Realizing activity is neither existent nor non-existent is our greatest challenge in the human form. We see phenomena all around us and believe them to be real. However, there is the Buddhist idea that none of the phenomena we see or experience are real. Rather, they are an expression of our karmic consequences and conditions. If this theory is true, what do we do when disease arises—cancer for exampe? Do we treat it or do we ignore it because it is not real anyhow? The correct answer is we treat it.

In order for the illusory, complex expression of karma to erupt, it must have a stage upon which to be expressed. Two venues exist for the purpose of such expression: conventional reality and ultimate reality. In conventional reality, people experience information through the five senses. This information is translated in our body and mind into some form of perception. In ultimate reality, phenomena appear, yet more like a movie—we watch it without reaction or response. We just let it be, and eventually it fades, like waves in the ocean.

We are constantly managing and navigating a phenomena-based reality and making decisions based on the phenomena. Making decisions about what shows up in our lives matters, and so does the nature of our responses to the phenomena. The tricky part is to avoid slipping down the rabbit hole of believing so harshly it is real, but instead to look at it as a much broader picture. Should cancer show up in your life, it does need to be treated. Allow the diagnosis to spark your investigation into the reasons the cancer manifested in the first place. Therein lies the opportunity for healing in the context of the phenomena-based reality.

How do we accept pain if our senses give us information, but that information is only essential to conventional reality? Many things that show up in the trajectory of life will grab our attention and instantly pull us into the present moment. In these cases, we experience the present moment in a deep, profound, and sometimes provocative way, not focused on the past or the future, but clearly situated in the present. Pain has a unique way of putting us in the present moment, unable to focus on our surroundings or environment clearly. It takes over the physical body and sometimes the emotional body in a profound and alarming manner, bringing us to our knees. When in acute pain, it can be impossible to think clearly or experience anything outside of the acuteness of the pain. If we could allow pain inside us, accept its volume of discomfort, it too is a teacher, a messenger, and a game-changer in our lives. Pain is easily one of the hardest sets of circumstances for humans to endure. Annoyance and aggravation can generally be tolerated by humans, especially in those who have experienced pain previously, and as long as it has an end point—childbirth, for example. However, severe injury causing acute and unmanageable pain that does not seem to have an end point is far more difficult to manage, accept, and experience its underlying provocation of the truth. The energy it requires is exhausting and the more common habit is to self-medicate in a desperate effort to make it stop.

Just as many topics discussed in this book mention operating on or across a continuum, so does pain. The pain scale varies from person to person because people are able to tolerate different degrees of pain and the current environment also dictates—for example, being shot in combat generally is accompanied by the benefit of adrenaline. The same is true in a shootout with police or a bad car accident. When pain reaches a point of unconsciousness or inability to function in daily activities, medication is and will be of great value. Once the pain has subsided, the greatest benefit is to evaluate the pain from an internal alchemical perspective, allowing the space for reflection and introspection.

What if we could allow an emotion such as anger to rise, and then just watch it; if we could refrain from repressing or oppressing the emotion, but act appropriately and let it move through us without impact? What if we could watch it arise, be in the present moment with it, and then just let it go, like waves in the ocean? We would feel the hurt, the pain, the anger, and then watch it leave, understanding it is nothing more than an eruption, a ripening, a moment of intense emotion, before it flees. If we humans could allow such a flow like a wave instead of holding on to our emotions and believing them to be "real," we might prevent the cancer from ever happening.

This idea suggests viewing our lives from a more objective platform in order to experience ourselves as happier and more content because we possess the understanding that activity is neither existent nor non-existent. It is simply the eruption and expression of our karmic consequences, and if we can make a decision, or respond to it as serene observers, we instantly alleviate the intense suffering it could otherwise impose.

The eight extraordinary vessels are mysterious, yet once embarked upon, understood, and accepted, they can open doors to a new existence. This work is about unblocking the mysteries of life, unleashing and accepting the pearls of life, and allowing for the bigger picture (lifetime to lifetime). The journey is unbelievable yet highly intellectual, but not literal; there is no dogma, and it is often described as drunk with the bliss of wisdom. Clearing the eight is a full-circle theory; moment to moment, it is critical in resolution of the karmic consequences of the individual for this life, then the next. The eight extraordinary vessels can be understood as a container to carry out the mission of the consciousness for the long haul until full enlightenment, not at the ego's judgment or opinion, but experienced as ultimate non-attachment, unconditional love that reverberates throughout and is felt by the masses in a way that is immeasurable and indescribable. Language becomes limited, useless, and unable to steer the course. Life becomes more pictorial and experiential. It is a journey, a trip, an evolution.

Bibliography

Baker, I. (1997) *The Tibetan Art of Healing*. London: Thames & Hudson.

Bercholz, S. and Kohn, S. (1993) *Entering the Stream*. Boston, MA: Shambhala Publications.

Chase, C. and Shima, M. (2010) *An Exposition on the Eight Extraordinary Vessels: Acupuncture, Alchemy, and Herbal Medicine*. Seattle, WA: Eastland Press.

Deadman, P., Al-Khafaji, M., and Baker, K. (2001) *A Manual of Acupuncture*. Hove: Journal of Chinese Medicine Publications.

Dechar, L. (2006) *Five Spirits: Alchemical Acupuncture for Psychological and Spiritual Healing*. New York, NY: Lantern Books.

Gyatso, T. (2015) *Essence of the Heart Sutra: The Dalai Lama's Heart of Wisdom Teachings*. Translated by Geshe Thupten Jinpa. Somerville, MA: Wisdom Publications.

Hammer, L. (1980) "The extraordinary acupuncture meridians: Homeostatic vessels." *American Journal of Acupuncture 8*, 2.

Hartman, D. (2011) *How the Eight Extraordinary Vessels Regulate the Heart Shen & Seven Emotions*. American Association of Acupuncture and Oriel Medicine Annual Conference.

Hicks, A., Hicks, J., and Hicks, P. (2004) *Five Element Constitutional Acupuncture*. Edinburgh: Elsevier Churchill Livingston.

Maciocia, G. (2005) *The Foundations of Chinese Medicine*. Edinburgh: Elsevier Churchill Livingston.

Matsumoto, K. (2012) *Kiiko Matsumoto Style of Acupuncture: Ren and Du Mai*. Workshop, Maryland Acupuncture Society.

Paulson, G. (2013) *Kundalini and the Chakras: Evolution in This Lifetime—A Practical Guide*. Woodbury, MN: Llewellyn Publications.

Santideva (7th century) *Bodhicaryavatara*. Translated by V. Wallace and B. Wallace (1997) *A Guide to the Bodhisattva Way of Life*. Ithaca, NY: Snow Lion Publications.

Sterman, A. (2012) *Advanced Acupuncture: A Clinic Manual*. New York, NY: Classical Wellness Press.

Tzu, Lao (4th century) *Tao Teh Ching*. Translated by J.C.H. Wu (2006) Boulder, CO: Shambhala Publication.

Veith, I. (trans.) (1949) *Huang Ti Nei Ching Su Wen: The Yellow Emperor's Classic of Internal Medicine*. Berkeley, CA: University of California Press.

Worsley, J.R. and Worsley, J.B. (2004) *Classical Five-Element Acupuncture, Volume 1 Meridians and Points* (4th edition). Portland, OR: Worsley Institute.

Zhen, Li Shi. (1518) *Bin Hu Mai Xue*. Translated by H. Huynh and G. Seifert (1985) *Pulse Diagnosis*. Brookline, MA: Paradigm Publications.

Zhibin, Z. and Unschuld, P. (2015) *Dictionary of the Ben Cao Gang Mu, Volume 1, Chinese Historical Illnesses Terminology*. Oakland, CA: University of California Press.

Index